Endocrinology

First and second edition authors:

Madeleine Dubuse

Stephan Sanders

Third edition authors:

Alexander Finlayson

Stephan Sanders

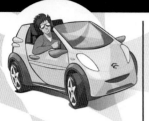

4th Edition
CRASH COURSE

SERIES EDITOR:

Dan Horton-Szar
BSc(Hons) MBBS(Hons) MRCGP
Northgate Medical Practice
Canterbury
Kent, UK

FACULTY ADVISORS:
Aftab Ahmad
Philip Weston
Consultant Diabetologist
Royal Liverpool University Hospital, Liverpool

Endocrinology

Ronan O'Neill
Fourth Year Student Doctor

Richard Murphy
Fourth Year Student Doctor

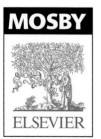

MOSBY

ELSEVIER

Edinburgh London New York Oxford Philadelphia St Louis Sydney Toronto 2012

ELSEVIER
MOSBY

Commissioning Editor: Jeremy Bowes
Development Editor: Catherine Jackson
Project Manager: Andrew Riley
Designer: Stewart Larking
Icon Illustrations: Geo Parkin
Illustration Manager: Jennifer Rose

First edition 1998

Second edition 2002

Third edition 2007

Fourth edition 2012

ISBN: 9780723436232

British Library Cataloguing in Publication Data
A catalogue record for this book is available from the British Library

Library of Congress Cataloging in Publication Data
A catalog record for this book is available from the Library of Congress

Notices
Knowledge and best practice in this field are constantly changing. As new research and experience broaden our understanding, changes in research methods, professional practices, or medical treatment may become necessary.

Practitioners and researchers must always rely on their own experience and knowledge in evaluating and using any information, methods, compounds, or experiments described herein. In using such information or methods they should be mindful of their own safety and the safety of others, including parties for whom they have a professional responsibility.

With respect to any drug or pharmaceutical products identified, readers are advised to check the most current information provided (i) on procedures featured or (ii) by the manufacturer of each product to be administered, to verify the recommended dose or formula, the method and duration of administration, and contraindications. It is the responsibility of practitioners, relying on their own experience and knowledge of their patients, to make diagnoses, to determine dosages and the best treatment for each individual patient, and to take all appropriate safety precautions.

To the fullest extent of the law, neither the Publisher nor the authors, contributors, or editors, assume any liability for any injury and/or damage to persons or property as a matter of products liability, negligence or otherwise, or from any use or operation of any methods, products, instructions, or ideas contained in the material herein.

 ELSEVIER your source for books, journals and multimedia in the health sciences

www.elsevierhealth.com

Working together to grow libraries in developing countries

www.elsevier.com | www.bookaid.org | www.sabre.org

ELSEVIER   **BOOK AID** International   Sabre Foundation

The Publisher's policy is to use **paper manufactured from sustainable forests**

Printed in China

Series editor foreword

The *Crash Course* series first published in 1997 and now, 15 years on, we are still going strong. Medicine never stands still, and the work of keeping this series relevant for today's students is an ongoing process. These fourth editions build on the success of the previous titles and incorporate new and revised material, to keep the series up to date with current guidelines for best practice, and recent developments in medical research and pharmacology.

We always listen to feedback from our readers, through focus groups and student reviews of the *Crash Course* titles. For the fourth editions we have completely re-written our self-assessment material to keep up with today's 'single-best answer' and 'extended matching question' formats. The artwork and layout of the titles has also been largely re-worked to make it easier on the eye during long sessions of revision.

Despite fully revising the books with each edition, we hold fast to the principles on which we first developed the series. *Crash Course* will always bring you all the information you need to revise in compact, manageable volumes that integrate basic medical science and clinical practice. The books still maintain the balance between clarity and conciseness, and provide sufficient depth for those aiming at distinction. The authors are medical students and junior doctors who have recent experience of the exams you are now facing, and the accuracy of the material is checked by a team of faculty advisors from across the UK.

I wish you all the best for your future careers!

Dr Dan Horton-Szar

Authors

The point of a medical textbook is to deliver clear and concise information on a specific field of medicine that is also clinically relevant. This new Crash Course Edition has been revised to focus more clearly on the topic of endocrinology and link the physiology to the disease processes in a more refined manner. The information on specific and highly relevant conditions, particularly diabetes, has been increased and the latest guidelines on management have been added. Other marked differences in this edition are also the removal of the excess of information on reproductive medicine and a change from MCQs and SAQs to the new Single Best Answer Questions, which are becoming more widely used by medical schools.

My hope is that this book will be of use to those beginning their medical education for forming the knowledge base that they will need in medicine, while being a revision tool for those who are already further along in the process.

Ronan O'Neill

As a medical student, endocrinology can be a difficult subject to fathom. There are numerous intricate systems and often complex terminologies that have to be understood and retained when studying. I hope that this edition of Crash Course Endocrinology will provide you with a reliable, concise and readable source of information whether you're new to the topic or you simply need some reassurance the night before your finals exam. Good luck!

Richard Murphy

Faculty Advisors

We live in exciting times in the world of diabetes and endocrinology. Our understanding of the diseases as well as our ability to manage the conditions have moved on enormously since the last edition of this book. Recent advances in the treatment of type 2 diabetes and the national guidelines around diabetes and endocrine conditions are all updated for this edition. With these developments and the limitations of space this edition concentrates on diabetes and endocrinology and old sections on pregnancy etc. have been dropped.

The two authors, both medical students, are to be congratulated on producing a guide to diabetes and endocrinology that should find a place on every medical and nursing students bookshelf. They have produced a book that provides not only informative text but also self-assessment questions to guide the learner.

Aftab Ahmad
Philip Weston

Acknowledgements

I think it's only fair that I start by thanking my partner in crime and co-author, Mr Richard Murphy. He was willing to take on the ridiculous task of helping to publish a medical textbook while still going through medical school.

I also want to thank Drs Weston and Ahmad who offered me this opportunity and then gave me the space to get on with the work until I needed them.

The next big thank you is to my mum, dad, brothers and, of course, my dog Max. They were there to encourage me the whole way with this book, which was at times the bane of my life and I can't thank them enough for it.

Now the acknowledgements get tricky, but in no particular order, I would like to thank my friends in Liverpool. Renee and Lisa who at this very moment are looking like a pair of zombies as we prepare for our exams. Also Asa and Fliss who put up with my whinging throughout the year.

Finally I'd like to thank all these other people for being there for me when I needed them. Brenndy Wright, Steve O'Hare, Tom, Paddy, Molly and everyone in the Liverpool Wilderness Medicine Society.

Ronan O'Neill

I would like to thank Ronan for giving me the opportunity to co-author this book. Special thanks to Verity, Jono and Owen for their continuous support and constant comedy over the past three years. I would also like to thank Drs Weston and Ahmed for their advice during the writing of the book.

Richard Murphy

Figure acknowledgements

Fig. 9.5 Reproduced with permission from R. Grainger and D. Allison, eds, Diagnostic Radiology: a textbook of medical imaging, 4th Edition, Churchill Livingstone, Elsevier

Figure 11.12 adapted from D Llewellyn-Jones, *Fundamentals of Obstetrics and Gynaecology*, 6th edition, 1994, by permission of Suzanne Abraham and Mosby.

Guidelines from NICE in Chapter 5: National Institute for Health and Clinical Excellence (2004) Adapted from 'CG 15 Type 1 diabetes: diagnosis and management of type 1 diabetes in children, young people and adults'. London: NICE. Available from http://www.nice.org.uk. Reproduced with permission.

Guidelines from NICE in Chapter 8: National Institute for Health and Clinical Excellence (2008) Adapted from 'TA 161 Alendronate, etidronate, risedronate, raloxifene, strontium ranelate and teriparatide for the secondary prevention of osteoporotic fragility fractures in postmenopausal women – Quick reference guide'. London: NICE. Available from http://www.nice.org.uk. Reproduced with permission.

Contents

Contents

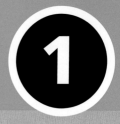

ROLE OF THE ENDOCRINE SYSTEM

The body requires a constant environment for cellular activities to take place. This is achieved by homeostasis, which is the process by which internal systems of the body are maintained within optimum parameters despite variations in external conditions. Homeostasis in the human body is controlled by the endocrine system, which uses chemical messengers called hormones to enable cellular communication and maintain this constant environment. Hormones are therefore vital in the coordination of virtually all body systems, both short term and long term.

Some short-term effects of the endocrine system include regulation of:

- Blood pressure
- pH of intracellular and extracellular fluids
- Respiration.

Some long-term effects include regulation of:

- Growth
- Reproduction
- Metabolism.

HORMONES AND ENDOCRINE SECRETION

What is a hormone?

The main function of hormones is to enable cells to communicate. There are five ways in which cells can communicate via hormones (Fig. 1.1):

- **Endocrine** – hormones are produced by an endocrine gland and transmitted by the circulatory system to alter the structure or function on target cells elsewhere in the body, e.g renin secreted by the kidney.
- **Paracrine** – hormones are produced by endocrine tissue and diffuse out of the cell to be transmitted through extracellular fluid to alter the structure or function of adjacent target cells. Distant cells are usually unaffected by paracrine hormones due to their low levels in the blood, e.g clotting factors in the blood.

- **Autocrine** – hormones are produced by a cell and act locally on the same cell, e.g. cytokines such as interleukin-1.
- **Neuroendocrine** – hormones are produced by specialized nerve cells and secreted from the nerve endings into the circulation. This is the boundary between the central nervous system and the endocrine system, e.g. oxytocin, ADH.
- **Neurocrine** – this does not strictly involve hormones but uses neurotransmitters to enable cell communication, e.g. serotonin. It causes specific, limited effects on target cells. There is some overlap between neurotransmitters and hormones, e.g. noradrenaline (norepinephrine) and adrenaline (epinephrine) are known as neurotransmitters when they cross synapses and hormones when there are released into the blood.

Types of hormone

Three classes of hormone are secreted into the blood:

- Polypeptides
- Steroids
- Modified amino acids.

Endocrine tissue

Endocrine tissue is simply tissue that secretes a hormone. These tissues respond to signals that either stimulate or inhibit the release of the specific hormone.

ORGANIZATION OF THE ENDOCRINE SYSTEM

The hypothalamus is an essential part of the endocrine system. It provides a link between the brain (central nervous system) and the rest of the body, allowing the brain to regulate body systems using hormones. The use of hormones to control peripheral organs and tissues allows a much wider range of effects compared to the specific, local effects of neurocrine communication. Hormones are required for coordinating long-term, sustained activities of multiple cells, tissues and organs. The peripheral tissues that hormones act on (Fig. 1.2), in

Overview of the endocrine system

Fig. 1.1   The routes by which chemical signals are delivered to cells.

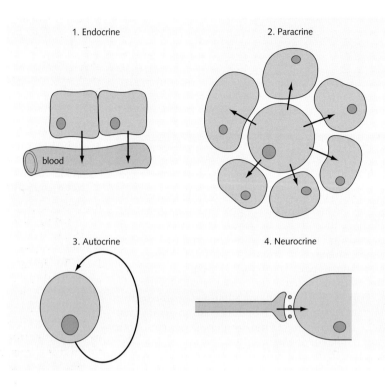

1. Endocrine

blood

2. Paracrine

3. Autocrine

4. Neurocrine

Fig. 1.2   The location of major endocrine organs and the hormones secreted by them.

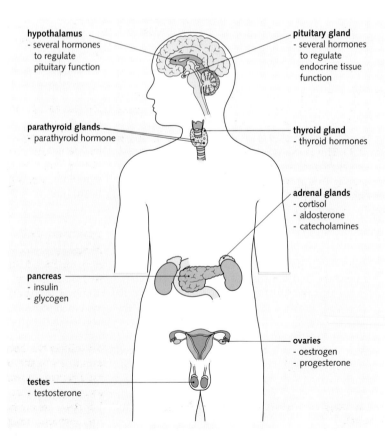

hypothalamus
- several hormones to regulate pituitary function

pituitary gland
- several hormones to regulate endocrine tissue function

parathyroid glands
- parathyroid hormone

thyroid gland
- thyroid hormones

adrenal glands
- cortisol
- aldosterone
- catecholamines

pancreas
- insulin
- glycogen

ovaries
- oestrogen
- progesterone

testes
- testosterone

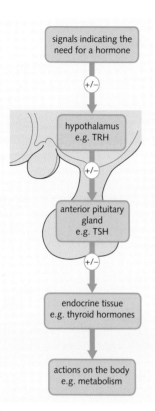

Fig. 1.3 The organization of the endocrine system (TRH, thyrotrophin-releasing hormone; TSH, thyroid-stimulating hormone).

constant environment for appropriate biochemical processes. If the equilibrium shifts, biochemical and neural signals converge on hypothalamic cells to provide negative feedback to the hypothalamus so it can make the necessary inhibitory or stimulatory adjustments to maintain homeostasis.

Hypothalamus

The hypothalamus is a structure located in the base of the forebrain. It converts neural signals received from the brain into chemical signals in the form of hormones. These hormones cause the release of other hormones in the pituitary gland. For this reason, hormones produced by the hypothalamus are known as 'releasing hormones', e.g. thyrotrophin-releasing hormone (from the hypothalamus) which causes the release of thyroxine in the pituitary gland. Releasing hormones therefore act indirectly on peripheral target cells; their actions are mediated through the release of pituitary hormones which have a direct effect on target cells.

Hypothalamic activity is altered by homeostatic signals (e.g. osmolarity of the blood) and sensory information arriving from the periphery (e.g. blood pressure, emotion). Hypothalamic hormones are released in a pulsatile manner, with regular changes in activity over the course of 24 hours (circadian rhythm). This change in activity over 24 hours corresponds to daily cycles of daylight and darkness and alters physiological processes such as body temperature, metabolic rate and blood pressure.

Pituitary gland

The pituitary gland is found at the base of the brain, inferior to the hypothalamus. It releases hormones into the blood in response to signals from the hypothalamus known as 'stimulating hormones'. Hormones from the pituitary gland regulate the function of peripheral endocrine tissues throughout the body.

Peripheral endocrine tissues

These tissues respond to signals from the pituitary by increasing or decreasing secretion of specific hormones into the blood. It is the hormones secreted by these peripheral tissues that affect the state of the body by acting on target cells.

turn, relay messages back to the hypothalamus about their effects and/or the levels of circulating hormones in the blood, and this causes either stimulation or inhibition of hormone release by the hypothalamus (Fig. 1.3). This is called negative feedback (Fig. 1.4).

The key to understanding the endocrine system is understanding that hormones produced by the hypothalamus alter the actions of peripheral endocrine tissues which act to restore equilibrium in order to maintain a

Target cells

All cells in the body will be exposed to the circulating hormones in the blood. The cell will only respond to the hormone, however, if it has the appropriate hormone receptor. Cells that are the intended object of action of a hormone are the hormone's target cell. There are multiple hormone receptors on every cell so the cell can

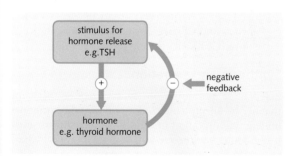

Fig. 1.4 Negative feedback (TSH, thyroid-stimulating hormone).

respond to different hormones. Target cells in different tissues may respond differently to the same hormone depending on the presence of certain receptors.

Control of hormone secretion

Overall control

Endocrine tissues are regulated by signals from a variety of neural and systemic sources. These signals are processed by cells to determine the rate of hormone secretion. The strength and importance of the signals varies so that hormone secretion fits the needs of the body.

> A single hormone may have multiple actions; equally, multiple hormones may have the same action. This is demonstrated by insulin and the regulation of blood glucose, respectively.

Neural control

Higher neural centres can influence the activity of the endocrine system by acting on the hypothalamus. They can increase or decrease the secretion of hypothalamic releasing hormones, which regulate the secretion of pituitary gland hormones. For example, cold external temperature will stimulate TRH, ultimately increasing metabolism in cells, raising body temperature.

Negative and positive feedback

A hormone is released in response to a stimulus. The actions of the hormone directly or indirectly reduce the intensity of the stimulus and restore equilibrium. Through this mechanism, homeostasis is achieved. This is known as negative feedback.

Hormones provide negative feedback:

Directly

The level of circulating hormones in the blood is detected by the hypothalamus or pituitary gland and subsequently altered, e.g. thyroxine levels are detected by the hypothalamus.

Indirectly

The actions of the hormone produce physiological effects which are detected and subsequently altered by the secretion of a hormone or hormones, e.g. low blood glucose levels (hypoglycaemia).

Feedback can also be positive, where the effect produced by a hormone promotes the stimulus that caused the release of the hormone. Positive feedback is not usually a homeostatic mechanism.

What are the benefits of having an endocrine system?

There are two main benefits to having an endocrine system:

Amplification

Subtle but important neural signals are detected by the hypothalamus, which then releases a small amount of 'releasing hormone'. The pituitary gland is able to secrete a greater quantity of 'stimulating hormone', which then stimulates the release of greater amounts of hormone by peripheral endocrine tissue. In this manner, the signal of a small number of neurons in the hypothalamus is amplified in three stages to affect the entire body.

Control

The endocrine system regulates all major body processes that are essential for life. These processes must be controlled very tightly and kept within normal physiological ranges or else death may occur. The complexity of the endocrine system allows such tight control and ensures the body can adapt and respond to any changes rapidly.

HORMONE TYPES AND SECRETION

Polypeptide hormones

Polypeptide hormones are proteins that act as hormones. They cannot pass through cell membranes due to their size and water-soluble nature. Protein hormones are the most abundant type of hormone (a safe bet in an exam). They are released by many structures including:

- Hypothalamus – TRH, GnRH, growth-hormone releasing hormone (GHRH), etc.
- Pituitary – TSH, follicle-stimulating hormone (FSH), luteinizing hormone (LH), oxytocin, etc.
- Pancreas and GI tract – insulin, glucagon, cholecystokinin (CCK), etc.

Synthesis and secretion

Polypeptide hormones are synthesized in the same manner as all proteins. Some polypeptide hormones undergo modification in the Golgi apparatus or secretory granules before secretion. Addition of carbohydrate groups to form glycoproteins is quite common as are cleavage reactions to free a smaller polypeptide hormone from the larger prohormone.

polypeptide-secreting cell

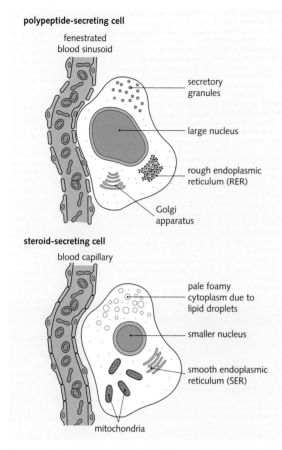

Fig. 1.5 Appearance of a polypeptide-secreting cell and steroid-secreting cell.

The secretory granules are released by exocytosis, in which the membrane of the granule fuses with the membrane of the cell causing the contents to be ejected. This process is triggered by calcium entering the cell.

Polypeptide hormone release is controlled mainly by regulating secretion of the hormone from the cell rather than synthesis (Fig. 1.5).

Lipid-derived hormones

These are divided into two categories:

- Steroid hormones – derived from cholesterol.
- Eicosanoids – derived from arachidonic acid, a phospholipid found in cell membranes.

Steroid hormones

Steroid hormones are small molecules that travel in the blood bound to plasma proteins since they are fat-soluble. Their solubility means they can cross cell membranes also. They are secreted by:

- **Adrenal cortex** – cortisol and aldosterone
- **Ovaries** – oestrogen and progesterone

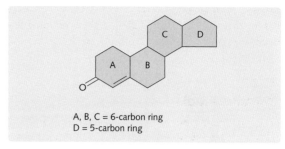

A, B, C = 6-carbon ring
D = 5-carbon ring

Fig. 1.6 Basic structure of a steroid hormone.

- **Placenta** – oestrogen and progesterone
- **Testes** – testosterone.

Synthesis and secretion

Steroids are derived from cholesterol by a series of reactions in the mitochondria and smooth endoplasmic reticulum. Cholesterol is acquired from the diet or synthesized within cells; it is stored in the cytoplasm of steroid cells (Fig. 1.5).

All steroids have the same basic structure formed by four rings of carbon (Fig. 1.6), but individual hormones differ in the following ways:

- Side chains attached to these rings
- Bonds within the rings (double or single).

The conversion of cholesterol into a steroid hormone is a two-step pathway:

Step 1
Cholesterol is converted into pregnenolone by the desmolase enzyme found within the mitochondria of steroid-producing cells.

Step 2
Pregnenolone is converted to progesterone by enzymes found in the mitochondria and cytoplasm. This reaction involves:

- Isomerization – the double bond moves from ring B to ring A.
- Oxidation – the hydroxyl group (OH) of ring A becomes a keto group (O).

Further steps are very variable, but the general pattern is shown in Fig. 1.7.

Steroid hormones are released immediately after synthesis so the rate of release is determined by the rate of synthesis, especially the synthesis of pregnenolone.

Eicosanoids

These are paracrine factors which regulate vital cell activities and enzymatic processes including immunity and inflammation. Arachidonic acid is broken down by

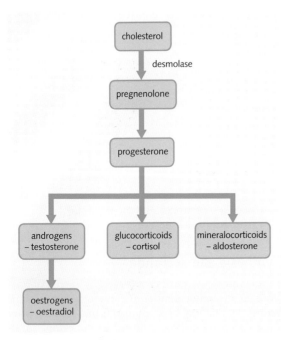

Fig. 1.7   Basic structure of a steroid hormone.

the enzyme phospholipase A_2. Two pathways create different groups of eicosanoids:

- Cyclooxygenase pathway – forms prostaglandins and thromboxanes
- Lipooxygenase pathway – forms leukotrienes.

Modified amino acids

These are small water-soluble hormones that can cross cell membranes.

Synthesis and secretion

These hormones are synthesized from the amino acids tyrosine and tryptophan.

Tyrosine derivatives
- Thyroid hormones from the thyroid gland
- Catecholamines (adrenaline and noradrenaline) from the adrenal medulla
- Dopamine from the hypothalamus.

Tryptophan derivatives
- Melatonin from the pineal gland
- Serotonin (5-HT) from GI tract, platelets and CNS.

The hormones are usually stored in secretory granules (except thyroid hormones, which are stored in follicles) and released by exocytosis in the same manner as polypeptide hormones. A comparison of the different types of hormone can be found in Figure 1.8.

HORMONE RECEPTORS

Hormone receptors are highly specific and are able to distinguish between hormones with very similar chemical structures. For example, testosterone and oestrogen have profoundly different effects on cells but are chemically very similar.

In order for a hormone to exert its effects on a cell, a hormone must interact with its appropriate receptor. There are two methods by which the hormone can interact with its receptor. This depends on whether the hormone is lipid-soluble (lipid derivatives) or water-soluble (polypeptides, amino acids) and therefore its ability to cross the cell membrane.

- Water-soluble hormones, which are unable to cross the cell membrane, use cell-surface receptors to exert

Fig. 1.8 Comparison of different types of hormone

	Polypeptides	Modified amino acids	Steroids
Size	Medium–large	Very small	Small
Ability to cross cell membrane	✕	✓	✓
Receptor type	Cell-surface	Cell-surface or intracellular	Intracellular
Soluble in:	Water	Water	Fat
Action	Protein activation	Protein activation or synthesis	Protein synthesis
Transport in the blood	Dissolved in the plasma	Dissolved in the plasma or bound to plasma proteins	Bound to plasma proteins

their effect on the cell. They activate or inhibit enzymes, which may affect protein synthesis.

- Lipid-soluble hormones, which are able to cross the cell membrane, use intracellular receptors to exert their effect on the cell, which usually involves control of gene expression. Lipid-soluble hormones and their intracellular receptors are utilized pharmaceutically due to their ability to be absorbed from the GI tract.

Hormones that act via cell-surface receptors can respond faster than those stimulating intracellular receptors because the activation of pre-existing enzymes takes less time than synthesizing new proteins. This explains why catecholamines released for the 'fight-or-flight' response use cell-surface receptors even though they can cross cell membranes.

A given hormone can have a different effect depending on the target cell and the receptor expressed on the cell membrane. Additionally, the number of receptors expressed by the cell can be increased or decreased to alter the strength of the hormone. This is known as 'up- and down-regulation' and affords the cell a limited degree of control, independent of circulating hormone concentrations.

- When hormone levels fall and the cell requires more of the hormone, the cell becomes more sensitive to the hormone by increasing the number of hormone receptors expressed. This is called up-regulation.
- When hormone levels rise and the cell requires less of the hormone, the cell becomes less sensitive by decreasing the number of hormone receptors expressed. This is called down-regulation.

Additionally, the receptor itself can become desensitized to circulating hormones. This is mediated by the hormone and involves phosphorylation of the receptor. The action is reversible. An example of this is adrenaline; a sustained stimulus (e.g. sky-diving) will produce a surge of catecholamines (e.g. adrenaline), which causes an initial rush, which then decreases despite the stimulus still being present.

Cell-surface receptors

Cell-surface receptors are utilized by polypeptide hormones and catecholamines. The receptor transmits the signal into the cell where it can have an effect. The cell-surface receptor spans the whole cell membrane so it has both an extracellular domain (for binding of hormones) and an intracellular domain (to allow the hormone signal to be relayed). This action is known as signal transduction.

There are two types of cell-surface receptor involved in the endocrine system:

- G-protein-coupled receptors (Fig. 1.9).
- Tyrosine kinase receptors (Fig. 1.10).

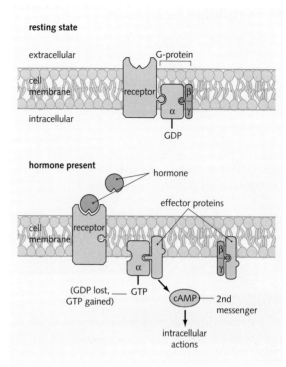

Fig. 1.9 Mechanism of action of a G-protein receptor (cAMP, cyclic adenosine monophosphate; GDP, guanosine diphosphate; GTP, guanosine triphosphate).

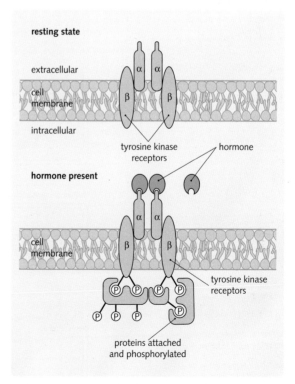

Fig. 1.10 Mechanism of action of a tyrosine kinase receptor.

Intracellular receptors

Hormones that readily cross the cell membrane, especially steroid hormones, use intracellular receptors. The receptors stimulate protein synthesis directly so they are also called transcription factors.

The hormone binds to the receptor in the cytoplasm, causing a change in shape that activates the receptor. The hormone and receptor then enter the nucleus where they bind to specific sections of DNA, stimulating or inhibiting the transcription of particular genes. This action alters protein synthesis in the cell, bringing about the intended effect of the hormone. This is shown in Fig. 1.11.

RELATIONSHIP OF THE NERVOUS AND ENDOCRINE SYSTEMS

Integration

The nervous and endocrine systems have a very close relationship, since they both use chemical signals to communicate between cells, and they may share a common evolutionary origin. The overlap between some hormones and neurotransmitters also supports this idea (e.g. somatostatin is found in both systems). The close relationship allows the two systems to coordinate responses to maintain homeostasis.

Neural control of hormones

The nervous system can control the endocrine system through two routes:

- Hypothalamus
- Autonomic nervous system (sympathetic and parasympathetic).

The endocrine system often acts as a long-term output from the brain to complement the action of short-term neural responses. This is demonstrated by the three responses to stress listed in the order they take effect:

- Noradrenaline is released from sympathetic nerves.
- Preformed adrenaline is released from the adrenal medulla.
- Cortisol is synthesized by the adrenal cortex.

Fig. 1.11 Mechanism of action of an intracellular receptor.

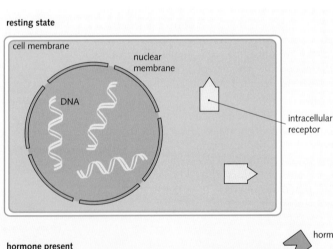

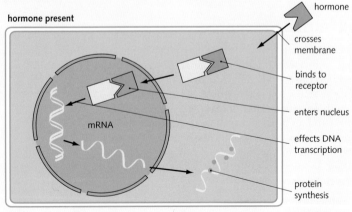

Hormonal control of neurons

To complete this circuit, the hormones of the endocrine system also affect the nervous system. Negative feedback to the hypothalamus has already been described. However, many hormones affect other areas of the brain, for example:

- Thyroid hormone deficiency causes depression.
- Leptin and insulin regulate feelings of hunger.
- Adrenaline increases mental activity.
- Melatonin regulates the feeling of tiredness.

Comparison between the nervous and endocrine systems

While the two systems function closely they have different modes of action. The hypothalamus combines these actions since it is an endocrine tissue composed of nerve cells called neurosecretory cells.

As endocrine hormones are very widespread in their distribution, the manifestations of endocrine disease vary greatly. Endocrine disease can be seen in patients of all ages, from congenital abnormalities in newborns through a plethora of adult and old-age endocrine problems. Patients with cancer can have endocrine dysfunction as part of the primary cancer (i.e. the cancer releases a hormone) or as a side effect of therapy. Endocrine disease can also occur in patients with infections, including HIV. Increasingly, associations are being demonstrated between endocrine disease and atherosclerotic cardiovascular disease. Therefore, the endocrine system is important to understand as it plays a key role in many other branches of medicine.

Nervous system

The nervous system uses very localized chemical signals at synapses to transmit membrane depolarization between neurons. The effects of the nervous system are very rapid but of short duration and expensive metabolically (i.e. the neurotransmitters and depolarization require a lot of energy). The specific target cell is determined mostly by the location of chemical release rather than the receptors.

Endocrine system

The endocrine system uses very generalized chemical signals, though a few endocrine tissues can depolarize. These signals require less energy than neural signals. The signals travel throughout the body in the bloodstream, and the target cell is determined mainly by the presence and specificity of receptors. The signals of the endocrine system tend to be slower but with a longer duration.

The hypothalamus and the pituitary gland

Objectives

By the end of this chapter you should be able to:
- Describe the function of the hypothalamic–pituitary axis
- Describe the embryological origin and anatomy of the hypothalamus and pituitary gland
- Name the pituitary hormones and the cells that secrete them
- Describe the aetiology of hypothalamic and pituitary gland disorders
- Recall the signs, symptoms, investigations and management of hypopituitarism and hyperpituitarism
- Differentiate between cranial and nephrogenic diabetes insipidus
- Describe the aetiology and clinical findings in SIADH.

The hypothalamic–pituitary axis is the central regulatory component of the endocrine system, consolidating signals from the brain, environmental stimuli and various feedback loops, adjusting output to meet changing demands.

The hypothalamus is sensitive to neural and hormonal stimuli. This information is then integrated by the hypothalamus to generate chemical signals that relay the message on to the pituitary. The hypothalamus is also sensitive to stimuli which affect hunger, thirst and sexual behaviour; however, the output of these stimuli is not the pituitary gland.

Hypothalamic-releasing and -inhibitory hormones are carried in the hypophyseal portal vessels to the anterior pituitary, where they regulate the release of anterior pituitary hormones.

The posterior pituitary gland functions in a slightly different way because it is a direct extension of the hypothalamus. Neurosecretory cells in the hypothalamus synthesize hormones that are transported along axons that terminate in the posterior pituitary. These hormones are then released into capillaries within the posterior pituitary gland to affect body parts directly.

ANATOMY

Hypothalamus

The hypothalamus is situated at the base of the forebrain, the diencephalon. Together with the thalamus, which is located superiorly, it forms the lateral walls of the third ventricle. It is posterior and slightly superior to the optic chiasm and anterior to the mamillary bodies. The inferior part of the hypothalamus – called the median eminence – gives rise to the pituitary stalk, which is continuous with the posterior pituitary gland.

The base of the hypothalamus between the median eminence and mamillary bodies is known as the tuberal area and contains nuclei which regulate pituitary gland function. This arrangement is shown in Fig. 2.2.

The hypothalamus receives multiple inputs about the homeostatic state of the body (Fig. 2.3). These arrive by two means:
- Circulatory, e.g. temperature, blood glucose, hormone levels
- Neuronal, e.g. autonomic function, emotional.

The ability of the hypothalamus to respond to circulatory stimuli is due to numerous connections to circumventricular organs which surround the ventricles of the brain. The hypothalamus also has extensive connections to sensory nuclei of the brainstem and limbic system which further modulate its activity (Fig. 2.4).

It responds to these inputs by secreting hormones that regulate the release of hormones from the anterior pituitary or releases hormones directly from the posterior pituitary.

The hypothalamus is composed of several components:
- Mamillary bodies – regulate feeding reflexes (e.g. swallowing) and memory
- Autonomic centres – control nuclei which alter heart rate and blood pressure
- Supraoptic nucleus – secretes ADH
- Tuberal nuclei – control of anterior pituitary
- Preoptic areas – control of thermoregulation
- Paraventricular nucleus – secretes oxytocin
- Suprachiasmatic nucleus – controls circadian rhythm.

Pituitary gland

The pituitary gland lies in a bony hollow of the sphenoid (the sella turcica), and it is covered by the fibrous diaphragma sellae. The optic chiasma lies directly

Fig. 2.1 Medial sagittal section of head showing the location of the hypothalamus and pituitary gland.

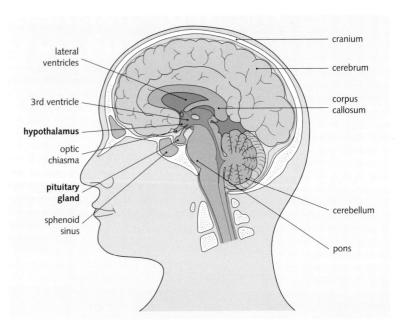

lateral ventricles

3rd ventricle

hypothalamus

optic chiasma

pituitary gland

sphenoid sinus

cranium

cerebrum

corpus callosum

cerebellum

pons

superior to the anterior pituitary. The posterior lobe is connected to the median eminence of the hypothalamus by the pituitary stalk (also known as the infundibulum).

The pituitary gland is divided into two lobes with distinct embryological origins, structure and function:

- Anterior pituitary (also known as adenohypophysis)
- Posterior pituitary (also known as neurohypophysis).

The cavernous sinuses, including cranial nerves III–VI, lie laterally (see Figs 2.1 and 2.2).

Blood supply

The superior hypophyseal arteries (branches of the internal carotid) form a capillary plexus around the median eminence, supplying blood to the hypothalamus. Hypothalamic hormones accumulate in the extracellular fluid at the median eminence before entering the capillary plexus. From here they enter hypophyseal portal vessels forming a portal circulation between the hypothalamus and anterior pituitary. The hypophyseal portal vessels terminate in a second capillary plexus in the anterior pituitary. This results in little dilution of hypothalamic hormones, allowing the pituitary to be closely regulated by small amounts of hypothalamic hormones. See Fig. 2.5.

The inferior hypophyseal arteries supply the posterior pituitary and do not communicate with the median eminence.

The cavernous sinuses drain the pituitary gland. This is how pituitary hormones enter the systemic circulation.

DEVELOPMENT

Hypothalamus

The hypothalamus develops from the embryological forebrain, specifically the diencephalon. It can be identified at week 6 of gestation.

Pituitary gland

The pituitary gland has two embryological origins:

- The infundibulum of the diencephalon which grows inferiorly. This is composed of neuroectoderm and forms the neurohypophysis. The neurohypophysis is therefore in direct communication with the hypothalamus. Axons from neurosecretory cells in the hypothalamus grow inferiorly into the pituitary stalk and terminate in the posterior pituitary gland.
- An outgrowth of the primitive oral cavity known as Rathke's pouch, which grows superiorly. This is composed of ectoderm and forms the adenohypophysis. The anterior pituitary is not in direct contact with the hypothalamus.

Rathke's pouch is visible from the third week of gestation and eventually loses its connection with the oral cavity and its blood supply at around the eighth week of gestation; the blood supply to the anterior pituitary is then replaced by hypothalamic portal vessels.

As the connection to the primitive mouth is lost, nests of epithelial cells may be left behind. Occasionally

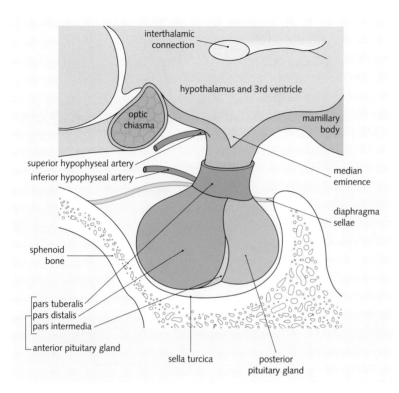

Fig. 2.2 Anatomical relationship of the pituitary gland and the hypothalamus to surrounding structures.

interthalamic connection

hypothalamus and 3rd ventricle

optic chiasma

mamillary body

superior hypophyseal artery
inferior hypophyseal artery

median eminence

diaphragma sellae

sphenoid bone

pars tuberalis
pars distalis
pars intermedia
anterior pituitary gland

sella turcica

posterior pituitary gland

Fig. 2.3 Inputs to the hypothalamus				
Circumventricular organs	**Limbic system**	**Nucleus of the solitary tract**	**Reticular formation**	**Olfactory system**
Monitor circulatory chemicals that normally have no access to the central nervous system. Include the organum vasculosum of the lamina terminalis (OVLT), which detects changes in osmolarity. Information from the OVLT is relayed, after processing in the hypothalamus, to the posterior pituitary, where ADH, the hormone that regulates blood osmolarity, is released.	The limbic system is responsible for emotion. It includes the amygdala (fear centre) and the hippocampus. Integration of these signals via the hypothalamus leads to endocrine responses to emotional changes, for instance sexual behaviour.	Conveys visceral sensory information, such as blood pressure (BP) and gut distension, which is important in the feedback control of BP/hunger/satiety.	Relays information from the spinal cord to the hypothalamus.	Conveys information about smell to the hypothalamus, which can initiate the endocrine and neural changes that lead to feeding responses such as salivation.

Fig. 2.4 The hypothalamic–pituitary system.

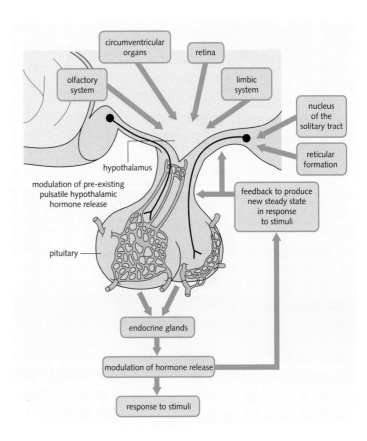

Fig. 2.5 Communication between the hypothalamus and pituitary gland; note the difference between the anterior and posterior pituitary gland.

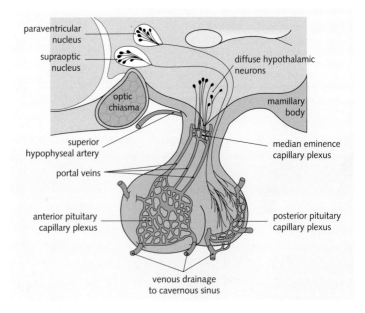

these cells are functional and secrete ectopic hormones (e.g. craniopharyngioma – see p. ••) but they are usually benign.

The embryology of the pituitary gland is shown in Fig. 2.6.

Soon after birth, the anterior pituitary gland begins to secrete gonadotrophins (LH and FSH) at roughly adult levels. Within 2 years, secretion declines rapidly to very low levels that are maintained until puberty. Sexual maturation is halted at this point.

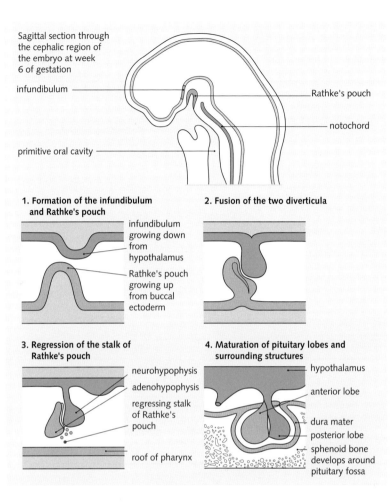

Fig. 2.6 Embryological development of the anterior and posterior lobes of the pituitary gland.

Sagittal section through the cephalic region of the embryo at week 6 of gestation

infundibulum

Rathke's pouch

notochord

primitive oral cavity

1. Formation of the infundibulum and Rathke's pouch

infundibulum growing down from hypothalamus

Rathke's pouch growing up from buccal ectoderm

2. Fusion of the two diverticula

3. Regression of the stalk of Rathke's pouch

neurohypophysis

adenohypophysis

regressing stalk of Rathke's pouch

roof of pharynx

4. Maturation of pituitary lobes and surrounding structures

hypothalamus

anterior lobe

dura mater

posterior lobe

sphenoid bone develops around pituitary fossa

MICROSTRUCTURE

Hypothalamus

There are a number of different secretory neurons in the hypothalamus (see p. ●●), each specialized to secrete specific hormones. Neurons that secrete the same hormones may be arranged in clusters called nuclei or they may be scattered diffusely.

Anterior pituitary

The anterior pituitary is composed of cords of secretory cells in a rich network of capillaries. Six types of secretory cell can be distinguished in the anterior pituitary (Fig. 2.7). They are listed along with the hormone(s) they secrete:

- Somatotrophs – growth hormone (GH)
- Gonadotrophs – luteinizing hormone (LH) and follicle-stimulating hormone (FSH)
- Corticotrophs – adrenocorticotrophic hormone (ACTH)
- Thyrotrophs – thyroid-stimulating hormone (TSH)
- Lactotrophs – prolactin
- Chromophobes – inactive secretory cells.

The anterior pituitary can be further divided into three parts, which have different secretory functions:

- Pars distalis: anterior portion of the adenohypophysis. This makes up the majority of the gland. It secretes GH, LH, FSH, ACTH, TSH and prolactin.
- Pars intermedia: a thin layer of corticotroph cells between the pars distalis and the posterior pituitary. It is poorly developed in humans. Secretes melanocyte-stimulating hormone (MSH) in the fetus and during pregancy.
- Pars tuberalis: surrounds the pituitary stalk. Contains a small number of mostly gonadotroph cells.

Posterior pituitary

The posterior pituitary can be divided into:

- Pars nervosa – majority of the posterior pituitary
- Pituitary stalk
- Median eminence.

Fig. 2.7 Hormones synthesized and secreted by the anterior pituitary and their effects

Hormone	Synthesized by	Stimulated by	Inhibited by	Target organ	Effect	Chapter
GH	Somatotrophs	GHRH	GHIH and IGF-1	Liver	Stimulates IGF-1 production and opposes insulin	9
TSH	Thyrotrophs	TRH	T_3	Thyroid gland	Stimulates thyroxine release	3
ACTH	Corticotrophs	CRH	Glucocorticoids	Adrenal cortex	Stimulates glucocorticoid and androgen release	4
LH+FSH	Gonadotrophs	GnRH, sex steroids	Prolactin, sex steroids	Reproductive organs	Release of sex steroids	11
Prolactin	Lactotrophs	PRF and TRH	Dopamine	Mammary glands and reproductive organs	Promotes growth of these organs and initiates lactation	11
MSH	Corticotrophs	–	–	Melanocytes in skin	Stimulates melanin synthesis in fetus and during pregnancy	–
Beta-endorphin	Corticotrophs	–	–	Unknown	May be involved in pain control	–

ACTH, adrenocorticotrophic hormone; CRH, corticotrophin-releasing hormone; FSH, follicle-stimulating hormone; GH, growth hormone; GHRH, growth-hormone releasing hormone; GnRH, gonadotrophin-releasing hormone; GHIH, growth-hormone inhibiting hormone; LH, luteinizing hormone; MSH, melanocyte-stimulating hormone; TRH, thyrotrophin-releasing hormone; TSH, thyroid-stimulating hormone.

The posterior pituitary is composed of two cell types but it contains no secretory cells:

- Non-myelinated axons, originating from the hypothalamus
- Pituicytes, which are glial support cells similar to astrocytes.

Within the axons, there are microtubules and mitochondria that are involved in the transport of neurosecretory granules. These granules travel from the hypothalamus to the axon terminals in the posterior pituitary, where they are stored before release. The axon terminals lie close to blood sinusoids, where the neurosecretory granules are released into the systemic circulation (Fig. 2.8).

HORMONES

Hormones of the hypothalamus

The hypothalamus secretes very small quantities of hormones into the portal veins to exert control over the anterior pituitary. By travelling in portal veins directly to the anterior pituitary, their concentration is high enough to produce an effect. The hypothalamic hormones are often released in a pulsatile manner. The pulses vary in amplitude and rate, often with a circadian rhythm (see Chapter 6). Hormones that influence the anterior pituitary are secreted by short parvocellular neurons. Hypothalamic neurons that travel directly to the posterior pituitary are magnocellular neurons.

Hormones that regulate anterior pituitary function

The hormones secreted by the hypothalamus are small peptides, except for dopamine, which is derived from the amino acid tyrosine. These hormones are shown in Fig. 2.9, along with their effects.

They act on the secretory cells of the anterior pituitary in an excitatory or inhibitory manner. Some peptide hormones have more than one action on anterior pituitary secretion, e.g. TRH stimulates prolactin release as well as TSH release.

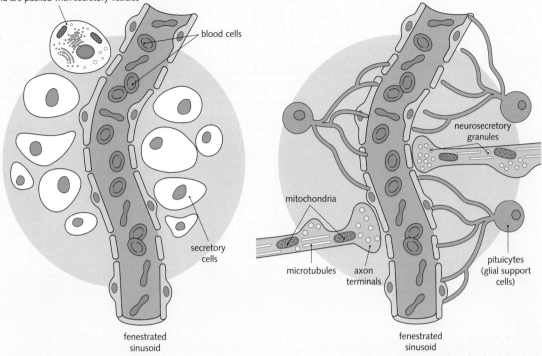

anterior pituitary

In common with all protein-secreting cells, the anterior pituitary cells contain abundant rough endoplasmic reticulum and Golgi bodies, and are packed with secretory vesicles

posterior pituitary

blood cells

secretory cells

fenestrated sinusoid

neurosecretory granules

mitochondria

microtubules   axon terminals

pituicytes (glial support cells)

fenestrated sinusoid

Fig. 2.8 Histology of the anterior and posterior pituitary gland.

Fig. 2.9 Hormones secreted by the hypothalamus and their effects on the secretion of the anterior pituitary hormones

Hormone	Target cells in the anterior pituitary gland	Effect on the anterior pituitary gland
Growth-hormone releasing hormone (GHRH)	Somatotrophs	↑ GH release
Growth-hormone inhibiting hormone (GHIH also called somatostatin)	Somatotrophs and thyrotrophs	↓ GH and TSH release
Corticotrophin-releasing hormone (CRH)	Corticotrophs	↑ ACTH release
Gonadotrophin-releasing hormone (GnRH)	Gonadotrophs	↑ LH and FSH release
Thyrotrophin-releasing hormone (TRH)	Thyrotrophs and lactotrophs	↑ TSH and prolactin release
Prolactin-releasing factors (PRF)	Lactotrophs	↑ Prolactin release
Dopamine (prolactin-inhibiting hormone)	Lactotrophs	↑ Prolactin release

ACTH, adrenocorticotrophic hormone; FSH, follicle-stimulating hormone; GH, growth hormone; LH, luteinizing hormone; TSH, thyroid-stimulating hormone.

Hormones released from the posterior pituitary

The small peptides ADH and oxytocin are synthesized in the cell bodies of magnocellular neurons arranged into two nuclei in the hypothalamus:

- Supraoptic nucleus
- Paraventricular nucleus.

Both nuclei secrete both hormones, but the supraoptic nucleus tends to secrete more ADH, whereas the paraventricular nucleus secretes more oxytocin. The hormones pass along the axons bound to glycoproteins. They pass through the median eminence where they are then stored before release.

Hormones of the anterior pituitary

The hormones secreted by the anterior pituitary are large peptides or glycopeptides. They are:

- Growth hormone (GH)
- Thyroid-stimulating hormone (TSH)
- Adrenocorticotropic hormone (ACTH)
- Luteinizing hormone (LH)
- Follicle-stimulating hormone (FSH)
- Prolactin (PRL).

The hormones synthesized by the anterior pituitary are released into the systemic circulation (Fig. 2.10).
They act in two ways:

- Regulation of other endocrine organs – TSH, ACTH, GH, LH and FSH
- Direct effects on distant organs – prolactin.

The pars intermedia of the anterior pituitary also secretes:

- α-MSH and γ-MSH, which stimulate melanocytes in skin in human fetal life and during pregnancy. Patients with high ACTH are hyperpigmented but it is unclear whether this is due to increased production of MSH or the melanotropic activity of ACTH.
- β-Endorphin, an endogenous opioid, which acts as a neurotransmitter and may have a role in the control of pain.

HORMONAL FEEDBACK

Hormones exert both positive and negative feedback on the hypothalamus. The hypothalamus then secretes releasing factors and inhibiting factors which affect pituitary hormone release. The pituitary gland also responds to feedback from circulating hormones and paracrine and autocrine secretions.

Hypothalamic regulation of prolactin release is unique because its action is inhibitory: dopamine secreted from the hypothalamus inhibits release of

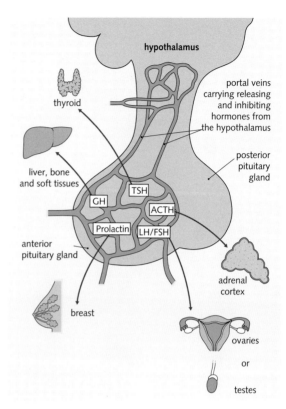

Fig. 2.10 Hormones of the anterior pituitary gland and their respective target organs. (ACTH, adrenocorticotrophic hormone; FSH, follicle-stimulating hormone; GH, growth hormone; LH, luteinizing hormone; TSH, thyroid-stimulating hormone.)

prolactin from the pituitary. This is important clinically if a tumour stops hypothalamic hormones from reaching the anterior pituitary. The levels of most pituitary hormones will fall, while levels of prolactin levels will rise. The use of dopamine antagonists in the treatment of psychiatric conditions commonly causes this effect also, causing galactorrhoea.

> The hormones of the anterior pituitary can be remembered using the mnemonic 'Fresh Pituitary Tastes Almost Like Guinness'.

Hormones of the posterior pituitary

Two major hormones are synthesized in the hypothalamus and released by the posterior pituitary into the systemic circulation:

- Antidiuretic hormone (ADH), also called arginine vasopressin (AVP)
- Oxytocin.

Fig. 2.11 Hormones secreted by the posterior pituitary and their effects

Hormone	Synthesized by	Stimulated by	Inhibited by	Target organ	Effect	Chapter
Antidiuretic hormone (ADH)	Supraoptic vasopressinergic neurons	Raised osmolarity; low blood volume	Lowered osmolarity, alcohol caffeine, glucocorticoids, ANF	Kidney	Increases the permeability of the collecting duct to reabsorb water	7
Oxytocin	Paraventricular oxytocinergic neurons	Stretch receptors in the nipple and cervix; oestrogen	Stress	Uterus and mammary glands	Smooth muscle contraction, leading to birth or milk ejection	13

Both are peptide hormones. Their main actions are shown in Figs 2.11 and 2.12.

Antidiuretic hormone

ADH acts mainly on the collecting ducts of the kidney to prevent water excretion. It also has a potent vaso-constricting action at high doses: hence the name vasopressin. Low blood volume detected by peripheral baroreceptors stimulates very high ADH release to increase blood pressure.

- V1A receptors are expressed by vascular smooth muscle and cause ADH's vasoconstrictive action.
- V2 receptors are expressed on the basolateral membrane of the distal convoluted tubule and collecting ducts of the kidney and are responsible for the hormone's antidiuretic effect.

A small proportion of ADH is released into the portal veins, where it stimulates corticotrophs in the anterior pituitary to secrete ACTH. This action is mediated via the V1B receptor (formerly known as V3 receptor).

Oxytocin

When a baby suckles the mother's breast, stretch receptors in the nipple send signals to the brain via sensory nerves. These signals reach the paraventricular neurons causing release of oxytocin from the posterior pituitary. The oxytocin reaches the myoepithelial cells of the breast, which contract, pushing milk out of the breast. This reflex is illustrated in Fig. •.••.

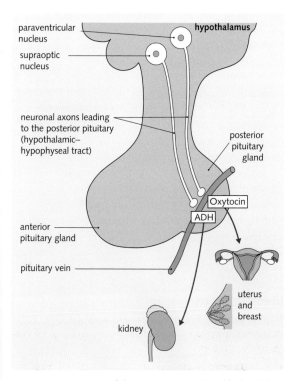

paraventricular nucleus
hypothalamus
supraoptic nucleus
neuronal axons leading to the posterior pituitary (hypothalamic–hypophyseal tract)
posterior pituitary gland
Oxytocin
ADH
anterior pituitary gland
pituitary vein
uterus and breast
kidney

Fig. 2.12 Hormones of the posterior pituitary gland and their respective target organs. (ADH, antidiuretic hormone.)

DISORDERS OF THE HYPOTHALAMUS

Primary diseases of the hypothalamus are very rare (approx. 1 in 50 000). They tend to cause deficiency of hypothalamic hormones and the corresponding pituitary hormones. Often, disorders of the hypothalamus can mimic pituitary pathology; however, the important distinction is that hypothalamic pathology often causes decreased secretion of most hormones but may cause increased secretion of some hormones, e.g. prolactin, as it is under inhibitory control by the hypothalamus.

The main causes of hypothalamic disorders are listed below:

- Trauma/surgery
- Radiotherapy
- Hormone excess – Syndrome of inappropriate antidiuretic hormone (SIADH), disconnection hyperprolactinaemia
- Hormone deficiency – Cranial diabetes insipidus, congenital gonadotrophin-releasing hormone (GnRH) deficiency (Kallmann's syndrome) causing infertility, congenital GHRH deficiency causing dwarfism
- Primary glial tumours of the hypothalamus.

Lesions in the hypothalamus can cause many other abnormalities including disorders of consciousness, behaviour, thirst, satiety and temperature regulation.

> In addition to endocrine abnormalities, pituitary tumours can present with the effects of a space-occupying lesion. These include headaches from stretching of the dura mater. Paradoxically, pituitary tumours can cause panhypopituitarism due to compression of functioning cells. Tumours of the pituitary gland are surrounded by the bone of the sella turcica, so they can only expand upwards into the optic chiasma, causing visual field defects. Further expansion compresses cranial nerves III, IV, V and VI in the wall of the cavernous sinus.

DISORDERS OF THE ANTERIOR PITUITARY

These can be grouped in a similar way to hypothalamic disorders:

- Hormone excess – Prolactin, GH (acromegaly), ACTH (Cushing's disease). These are most commonly due to benign tumours of the secretory cells called pituitary adenomas. TSH, LH and FSH adenomas are rare. Functioning adenomas usually present whilst small and cause disease by excess hormone release.
- Hormone deficiency – Hypopituitarism or compression by a space-occupying lesion (e.g. adenoma). Non-functioning adenomas usually present later as a macroadenoma and cause disease by compressing surrounding structures. This frequently causes insufficient pituitary hormone release either by compression of the portal vessels or secretory cells.

Pituitary tumours can present in a number of ways:

- Headache and visual disturbance from compression
- Inappropriate hormone secretion, e.g. prolactin (hyperprolactinaemia), ACTH (Cushing's disease), GH (acromegaly)

- Hormone hypo- or hypersecretion due to compression
- Amenorrhoea and/or loss of libido.

Hyperpituitarism

All anterior pituitary cells are capable of becoming neoplastic (Fig. 2.14). They are usually classified according to their location, size and invasiveness:

- Microadenomas – tend to be intrasellar and are < 10 mm in diameter. These are more common than macroadenomas.
- Macroadenomas – are > 10 mm in diameter and tend to compress adjacent structures.

Between 10 and 20% of the population have pituitary microadenomas, which are clinically silent.

Prolactinomas

Prolactinomas are the most common functioning adenoma of the anterior pituitary gland. They are more common in women and tend to present early, with oligomenorrhoea, amenorrhoea and infertility. Galactorrhoea may occur as a result of excess prolactin secretion by the adenoma.

Prolactinomas may present differently in men, with erectile dysfunction, visual field defects and headache (Fig. 2.15).

Hyperprolactinaemia may also be caused by some medications.

Infertility is the result of prolactin interfering with the release of GnRH, which inhibits LH and FSH release and causes hypogonadism.

> Prolactin-secreting adenomas are the most common type of functioning adenoma and secrete excess prolactin by definition. Hyperprolactinaemia and galactorrhoea can also be caused by dopamine antagonists used to treat patients with movement disorders. Furthermore, renal failure can be associated with hyperprolactinaemia due to impaired prolactin secretion. Non-functioning adenomas can also produce hyperprolactinaemia by removing dopaminergic inhibition of prolactin release.

Investigations

A number of symptoms and investigations are assessed to achieve a diagnosis:

- Visual field assessment is carried out to detect compression of the optic chiasma which presents as bitemporal hemianopia. Diplopia may also be present as a result of cavernous sinus involvement.

Are there abnormal hormone levels in the blood? Serum levels of the following hormones should be analysed, ideally in the morning, as this will give you a clinical picture of what pathology is under way:

- Prolactin
- TSH and thyroxine
- Insulin-like growth factor 1
- FSH, LH and levels of oestrogen/testosterone
- ACTH and cortisol.

Magnetic resonance imaging (MRI) or computed tomography (CT) scans are used to detect abnormal anatomy. Radiolabelled dopamine receptor antagonists can also aid visualization of prolactinomas.

Suppression tests may also be carried out to assess pituitary response to hormone analogues or inhibiting factors to locate the lesion on the endocrine axis. Generally, adenomas display reduced negative feedback.

Suppression tests are used to determine if anterior pituitary secretion is still controlled by negative feedback. The main suppression tests for anterior pituitary levels are to measure:

- GH in response to an oral glucose tolerance test, which normally suppresses GH levels
- ACTH in response to dexamethasone, a steroid that normally suppresses CRH and ACTH release.

Treatment

There are four methods of treating excess hormone production, but they all carry the risk of causing hypopituitarism:

- Bromocriptine (dopamine agonist) to reduce prolactin secretion
- Octreotide (synthetic somatostatin) to reduce GH secretion
- Surgical removal of pituitary adenoma
- Irradiation to prevent adenoma recurrence.

Surgery on the pituitary gland is indicated when the lesion is causing compression of surrounding structures or when medical treatment has been unsuccessful.

Irradiation is indicated for persistent hypersecretion of pituitary hormones, or when surgery is contraindicated.

Hypopituitarism

Pituitary insufficiency (hypopituitarism) often presents with insidious-onset depression, tiredness and hypogonadism. Panhypopituitarism refers to a deficiency of all anterior pituitary hormones. The causes of pituitary insufficiency are more varied than those of hyperpituitarism. However, the most common cause is treatment of hyperpituitarism.

Non-functioning adenomas

These are the most common type of pituitary tumour and do not produce hormones. They are most commonly non-functioning gonadotroph cells. Since there is no excess hormone production they usually present late with symptoms caused by compression of surrounding structures. Symptoms are usually progressive:

- Headache, vomiting and papilloedema due to raised intracranial pressure
- Visual disturbance
- Oligomenorrhoea and amenorrhoea in women
- Reduced libido and infertility in men
- Cranial nerve palsies.

The tumour can cause hormone deficiencies by direct compression of the secretory cells or by compressing the portal veins that bring the hypothalamic-releasing factors. Secretion of anterior pituitary hormones is inhibited in a characteristic order: GH, LH, FSH, ACTH, TSH, prolactin (see Fig. 2.13). Unless the compression is severe, prolactin secretion often increases (see p. ••).

Other tumours

Tumours in surrounding tissues can also compress the pituitary gland, causing hypopituitarism, the most common being:

- Craniopharyngiomas
- Gliomas (especially in the optic chiasm)
- Meningiomas
- Metastases (particularly from breast, bronchus and kidney).

Craniopharyngiomas are tumours arising from remnants of Rathke's pouch. Occasionally they are functional and secrete ectopic hormones but they are usually benign. They are rare but are the most common intracranial tumour affecting children. Hypothalamic symptoms predominate and can be varied. Children usually present with growth failure.

Gliomas are primary tumours of the glial support cells.

Meningiomas are formed from arachnoid and meningioendothelial cells. They are usually highly vascular and consequently carry a high risk of haemorrhage during surgery.

Infarction of the pituitary gland

Infarction of the pituitary gland causes necrosis of all secretory cells with resultant panhypopituitarism, including loss of prolactin secretion. Sheehan's syndrome is a rare cause of pituitary infarction, which is caused by hypotension and/or hypovolaemic shock during obstetric haemorrhage. The pituitary gland enlarges during pregnancy and becomes highly vascular as a result; therefore it is particularly susceptible to hypotension and hypoxia. The ensuing panhypopituitarism causes

Fig. 2.13 Anterior pituitary hormones and the disorders caused by their deficiency and excess

Hormone	Deficiency	Excess
GH	Dwarfism in children or adult GH deficiency syndrome	Gigantism in children, acromegaly in adults
LH and FSH	Gonadal insufficiency (decreased sex steroids)	Extremely rare but causes infertility
ACTH	Adrenocortical insufficiency (decreased cortisol and adrenal androgens)	Cushing's disease (increased cortisol and adrenal androgens)
TSH	Hypothyroidism (decreased thyroid hormones)	Extremely rare but causes hyperthyroidism (increased thyroid hormones)
Prolactin	Hypoprolactinaemia (failure in postpartum lactation)	Hyperprolactinaemia (impotence in males, amenorrhoea in females and decreased libido)

ACTH, adrenocorticotrophic hormone; FSH, follicle-stimulating hormone; GH, growth hormone; LH, luteinizing hormone; TSH, thyroid-stimulating hormone.

Fig. 2.14 Adenomas of the anterior pituitary gland and their effects

Tumour	Hormone excess	Percentage of all pituitary tumours	Disease	Chapter
Prolactinoma	Prolactin	50%	Hyperprolactinaemia	2
Non-secretory prolactinoma	None	20%	Hypopituitarism	2
Somatotrophic cell adenoma	GH	20%	In children: gigantism In adults: acromegaly	9
Corticotrophic cell adenoma	ACTH	5%	Cushing's disease	4
Gonadotrophic cell adenoma	LH and FSH	Very rare	Infertility	–
Thyrotrophic cell adenoma	TSH	Very rare	Hyperthyroidism	3

ACTH, adrenocorticotrophic hormone; FSH, follicle-stimulating hormone; GH, growth hormone; LH, luteinizing hormone; TSH, thyroid-stimulating hormone.

a failure to lactate, amenorrhoea and eventually death if untreated.

Pituitary apoplexy is a rare endocrine emergency which is caused by infarction or haemorrhage of a pituitary tumour. The most common precipitants of pituitary apoplexy are hypertension and major surgery. Patients typically present with the following:

- Sudden-onset severe headache (thunderclap). This is classically retro-orbital

- Nausea, vomiting and decreased conscious level
- Ophthalmoplegia (paralysis or weakness of one or more extraocular muscles)
- Sudden severe visual impairment or loss. Bitemporal hemianopia is the most common visual field defect seen.

These signs and symptoms are usually followed by a deficiency of one or more anterior pituitary hormones. The most common anterior pituitary hormone to be

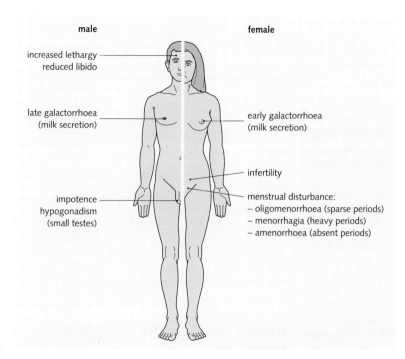

male

increased lethargy
reduced libido

late galactorrhoea
(milk secretion)

impotence
hypogonadism
(small testes)

female

early galactorrhoea
(milk secretion)

infertility

menstrual disturbance:
– oligomenorrhoea (sparse periods)
– menorrhagia (heavy periods)
– amenorrhoea (absent periods)

Fig. 2.15 Symptoms and signs of hyperprolactinaemia. Women tend to present earlier with endocrine symptoms.

lost is ACTH, which can lead to acute secondary adrenal insufficiency. Investigations include:

- Electrolytes
- Pituitary hormones
- Glucose
- MRI (or if unavailable CT).

To counteract haemodynamic instability, high-dose IV hydrocortisone should be given. Transsphenoidal surgical decompression should be performed within one week and is generally reserved for patients with:

- Severe neuro-ophthalmic signs
- Deteriorating conscious level.

Compression of the pituitary gland

Empty sella syndrome is a condition where the sella turcica partially or completely fills with cerebrospinal fluid. The majority of patients have no associated pituitary problems, but it may cause pituitary compression, which could lead to pituitary insufficiency. It is not always pathological.

Other causes of pituitary failure

Pituitary failure can also be caused by inflammatory/infiltrative processes, e.g. sarcoidosis, lymphocytic hypophysitis, haemochromatosis and infective processes, e.g. TB and syphilis.

Diagnosis of hypopituitarism

Diagnosis of hypopituitarism involves the same steps as for hyperpituitarism; however, stimulation tests are used instead of suppression:

- Visual field assessment
- Basal hormone levels in the blood
- Stimulation tests
- MRI or CT scan.

The main stimulation tests for anterior pituitary levels are to measure:

- GH in response to an insulin tolerance test, which normally increases GH levels
- Cortisol in response to hypoglycaemia or the ACTH analogue Synacthen
- LH and FSH in response to GnRH or the anti-oestrogen clomifene.

Treatment of hypopituitarism

The main treatment of hypopituitarism is hormone replacement, which requires frequent monitoring. All major anterior pituitary hormones can be replaced, though prolactin is not readily available since it is rarely needed:

- Subcutaneous GH replacement using human recombinant GH. This is only indicated for severe GH deficiency which is severely affecting the patient's quality of life
- Oral thyroxine once cortisol replacement has begun

- Oral or intramuscular testosterone in males
- Oral oestrogen and progesterone cyclically in females
- Intramuscular human chorionic gonadotrophin, LH and FSH for infertile males and females.

DISORDERS OF THE POSTERIOR PITUITARY

Diabetes insipidus

Diabetes insipidus is the name for the pathological state in which large amounts of hypotonic, dilute urine are passed (polyuria). This leads to excessive thirst (polydipsia). It is due to either a deficiency of ADH secretion (cranial diabetes insipidus), or an inappropriate renal response to ADH (nephrogenic diabetes insipidus). As a result, fluid reabsorption at the kidneys is impaired causing the characteristic signs and symptoms. Up to 20 litres of water can be passed in a day, causing potentially fatal dehydration (particularly in unconscious patients) and persistent thirst.

Diabetes insipidus is often diagnosed according to the clinical history in addition to elevated plasma osmolality (>300 mOsm/kg), and low urine osmolality (<600 mOsm/kg).

Hyperglycaemia, hypercalcaemia and hypokalaemia should be ruled out.

An ADH stimulation test is used to distinguish between cranial diabetes insipidus and nephrogenic diabetes insipidus:

- Cranial diabetes insipidus is illustrated by an inability to concentrate urine after fluid restriction alone, but the ability to concentrate urine after administration of ADH.
- Nephrogenic diabetes insipidus shows an inability to concentrate urine even after administration of ADH.

Fig. 2.16 Posterior pituitary hormones and the disorders caused by their deficiency and excess

Hormone	Deficiency	Excess
ADH	Diabetes insipidus (polyuria, hypotension)	Syndrome of inappropriate ADH secretion (SIADH)
Oxytocin	Failure to progress in labour and difficulty with breastfeeding	No effect

ADH, antidiuretic hormone.

The condition is treated with desmopressin, a long-acting vasopressin analogue.

Some medications can also alter ADH levels.

Excess antidiuretic hormone secretion

The syndrome of inappropriate antidiuretic hormone secretion (SIADH) can be caused by neurological, endocrine, malignant or infective diseases, but it can also be idiopathic, postoperative or caused by medications. Excess ADH secretion causes water retention resulting in hypo-osmotic hyponatraemia (low plasma sodium).

Patients will have:

- Hyponatraemia
- Low plasma osmolality
- High levels of urinary sodium
- High urine osmolality.

Additionally, patients are euvolaemic (normal blood volume) and normotensive (normal blood pressure).

The symptoms progress from malaise and weakness to confusion and coma. If untreated, it can be fatal. Oedema does not occur (see Fig. 2.16).

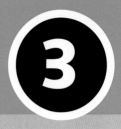
Objectives

By the end of this chapter you should be able to:
- Explain the structure and development of the thyroid gland
- Describe the synthesis of thyroid hormones
- Understand the regulation and physiological effects of thyroid hormones
- Discuss the major disorders associated with thyroid function.

The thyroid gland is the largest endocrine organ in the body and is tasked with regulating the metabolism of most of the body's cells. It also plays a vital role in the development of the nervous and skeletal systems. The gland is located anterior to the trachea on the lower aspect of the neck and is composed of two lobes joined by a piece of tissue called the 'isthmus'.

The gland contains a large store of preformed thyroid hormones arranged in microscopic spherical sacs called thyroid follicles. It also acts as a large iodine store, as the production of thyroid hormones is dependent on adequate iodine being available. The release of thyroid hormones (Fig. 3.1) is regulated by the anterior pituitary gland, which secretes thyroid-stimulating hormone (TSH). The two hormones secreted by the follicles are:

- T_4 – a prohormone that acts as a plasma reservoir
- T_3 – the active hormone.

Hyperthyroidism is the excessive release of thyroid hormones resulting in an abnormally raised metabolism. This classically presents with the patient feeling hot and sweaty and complaining of unexplained weight loss.

Hypothyroidism is the deficient release of thyroid hormone resulting in an abnormally low metabolism. The patient will complain of feeling lethargic and cold, with unexplained weight gain.

ANATOMY

Thyroid gland

The thyroid gland is butterfly-shaped and located inferior to the larynx and cricoids cartilage. It has two pyramidal-shaped lateral lobes, approximately 5 cm in long, joined by the narrower isthmus anterior to the trachea. It is usually located over the second and third tracheal cartilages (Fig. 3.2).

The thyroid is attached to the trachea by the pretracheal fascia (Fig. 3.3) so that it moves with the trachea and larynx when swallowing but not when the tongue is protruded. The thyroid is covered by a fibrous capsule within the fascia.

Blood, nerves and lymphatics

The thyroid is highly vascularized, receiving 80–120 mL of blood per minute. The vascular supply to the thyroid comes from the superior and inferior thyroid arteries; however, a small percentage of people have a third artery that supplies the isthmus, called the thyroid ima artery.

1. The **superior thyroid artery** is the first branch of the external carotid artery and it descends to the superior point of the gland's lateral lobe. When it reaches the gland, the artery divides into the anterior and posterior glandular branches. The **anterior glandular branch** passes along the superior border of the gland and anastomoses with its twin from the opposite side. The **posterior glandular branch** passes to the posterior side of the gland.
2. The **inferior thyroid artery** is a branch of the thyrocervical trunk that arises from the first part of the subclavian artery. It ascends passing posterior to the carotid sheath, and reaches the lateral lobe of the gland at the inferior pole. The inferior thyroid artery divides into two branches, the inferior branch and ascending branch. The **inferior branch** supplies the lower part of the thyroid gland and anastomoses with the posterior branch of the superior thyroid artery. The **ascending branch** supplies the parathyroid glands.
3. The **thyroid ima artery** is small and not always present. It can arise from two possible locations, the arch of the aorta or the brachiocephalic trunk, from which it ascends to the anterior surface of the trachea to supply the thyroid gland.

The thyroid gland is drained by three veins:

- The **superior thyroid vein**, which drains the area supplied by the superior thyroid artery

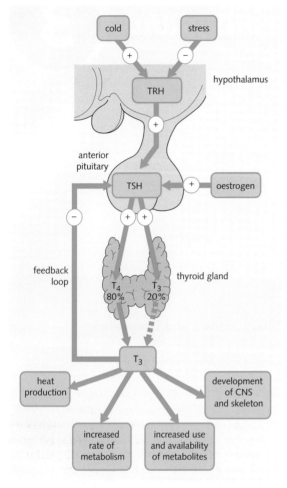

Fig. 3.1 Hormonal regulation of the thyroid hormones. (T_3, triiodothyronine; T_4, thyroxine; TRH, thyrotrophin-releasing hormone; TSH, thyroid-stimulating hormone.)

- The **middle** and **inferior thyroid veins**, which drain the rest of thyroid gland.

The superior and middle thyroid veins drain into the internal jugular vein and the inferior thyroid vein drains into the brachiocephalic vein.

Thyroid lymphatics drain into four groups of nodes:

- Prelaryngeal lymph nodes
- Pretracheal lymph nodes
- Paratracheal lymph nodes
- Deep cervical lymph nodes.

Parathyroid glands

The parathyroid glands are two pairs of small, oval structures approximately 5 mm in diameter, one pair located on the posterior surface of each lobe. The glands are designated as the inferior and superior pairs.

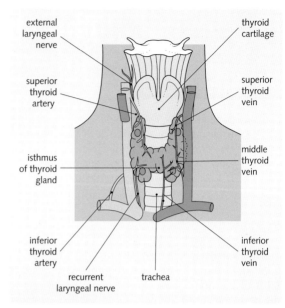

Fig. 3.2 View of the neck, showing the location and blood supply of the thyroid gland.

However, it is important to note that the number of glands can vary, as can their location. The function of the parathyroid glands is described in Chapter 8.

MICROSTRUCTURE

Thyroid gland

The thyroid is composed of approximately one million microscopic spherical follicles. The wall of each follicle is made up primarily of epithelial cells, called follicular cells. These cells surround and extend into a colloid-filled space. The follicular cells secrete thyroglobin, a storage form of thyroid hormone, into the colloid. When the follicular cells are not actively secreting hormones, their shape is low cuboidal to squamous, but when under the influence of TSH they become cuboidal or low columnar and actively secrete hormones. The colloid store and follicles increase in size when they are not carrying out active secretion of hormones.

When the follicular cells are in an active secretory phase, microvilli form on their inner surface and thyroglobin is absorbed. This results in the colloid store shrinking in size. The thyroglobin is broken down in the cell and released as thyroid hormone. The histology of the thyroid gland is shown in Fig. 3.4.

Another type of secretory cell is located on the follicles, within the basement membrane that surrounds the follicles. These are called parafollicular cells (C cells), which synthesize and secrete calcitonin.

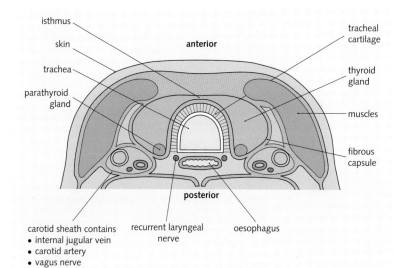

Fig. 3.3 Horizontal section of the anterior neck at the level of the sixth cervical vertebra, showing the location of the thyroid and parathyroid glands and their surrounding structures.

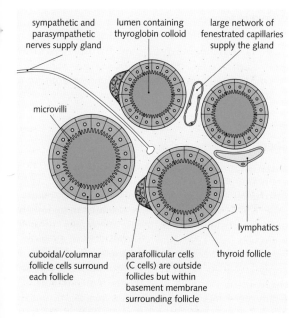

Fig. 3.4 Histology of the thyroid gland.

Parathyroid glands

The parathyroid glands are composed of two types of epithelial cells:

- **Chief (principal) cells** – synthesize parathyroid hormone (PTH), also known as parathormone
- **Oxyphil cells** – exhausted chief cells that increase in number with age. They have no known function.

DEVELOPMENT

Thyroid gland

The thyroid develops in the fourth week as a midventral outgrowth of endoderm from the floor of the pharynx, named the **thyroid diverticulum**. It moves inferiorly into the neck and differentiates into the lateral lobes and isthmus of the thyroid gland. The gland remains attached to the tongue by the thyroglossal duct.

Approximately half the population have a remnant of this duct, in the form of a small pyramidal lobe that extends superiorly from the isthmus. This is important because thyroglossal cysts can form anywhere along the thyroid's course, presenting as neck lumps that rise when the tongue is protruded.

Parathyroid gland

The parathyroid glands develop from the endoderm, at the level of the third and fourth pharyngeal pouches. The dorsal portion of the third pouch forms the inferior parathyroid glands, while the superior pair of glands are formed by the dorsal portion of the fourth pouch.

THYROID HORMONES

The thyroid gland is unique amongst the endocrine glands because it stores large quantities of its secretory product (approximately 100 days worth). This means that deficiency can take a while to present clinically.

Three hormones are synthesized and secreted in the gland:

- Thyroxine (T_4)
- Tri-iodothyronine (T_3)
- Calcitonin.

Calcitonin is involved in calcium homeostasis and is discussed in Chapter 8.

Synthesis

T_3 and T_4 are derived from two molecules of the amino acid and iodine. T_3 contains three iodine atoms and T_4 contains four. There structures are shown in Fig. 3.5.

The synthesis of thyroid hormones occurs in the follicle lumen. The process of T_3 and T_4 synthesis involves the processing of tyrosine and iodine, followed by a reaction to bind them together. These steps are shown in Fig. 3.6.

Tyrosine processing is relatively simple since tyrosine molecules are already within the cell.

Thyroglobulin synthesis

- Tyrosine is converted into the glycoprotein thyroglobulin, which contains approximately 110 tyrosine residues.

The processing of iodine involves two stages as plasma iodine concentrations are very low.

Iodine trapping

- Plasma iodide ions (I^-) are actively transported from the plasma into the follicular cells against a steep concentration gradient. This is a rate-limiting step.

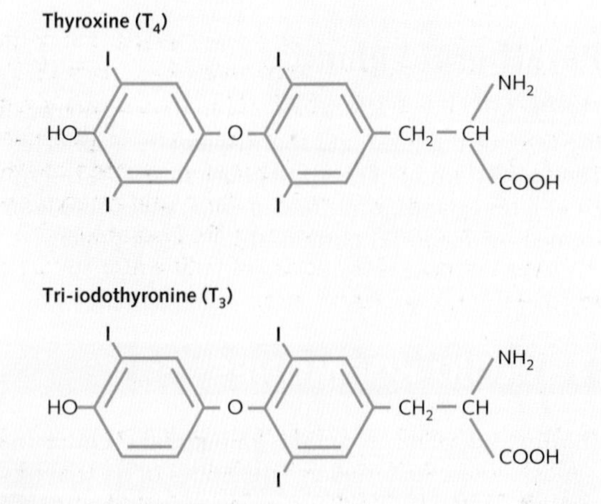

Thyroxine (T_4)

Tri-iodothyronine (T_3)

Fig. 3.5 Structures of T_3 and T_4.

Iodide oxidation

- Iodide is rapidly oxidized to iodine (I_2) by hydrogen peroxide, a reaction catalysed by a haem-containing enzyme, thyroid peroxidase (TPO). TPO is located on the luminal surface of follicular cell membrane.

The two components are then combined in the colloidal lumen.

Iodination of thyroglobulin

- Reactive iodine rapidly attaches to the tyrosine molecules within the extracellular thyroglobulin. The reaction is catalysed by TPO, and monoiodotyrosine (MIT or T_1) and diiodotyrosine (DIT or T_2) are formed.

Coupling

- Once tyrosine is iodinated, it is taken up into the thyroglobulin colloid of the follicle and coupled together. Combinations of T_1 and T_2 can form thyroid hormones:

  - T_3 (tri-iodothyronine) is made from $T_1 + T_2$
  - T_4 (tetra-iodothyronine or thyroxine) is made from $T_2 + T_2$.

  Only a small proportion of coupling reactions form T_3 and T_4. Thyroid hormones are now available for release on demand.

Secretion

This is controlled by thyroid-stimulating hormone (TSH or thyrotrophin). Under the influence of TSH, iodinated thyroglobulin is taken into the follicular cells by pinocytosis. This fuses with lysosomes, resulting in hydrolysis of the thyroglobulin and release of coupled tyrosine molecules (e.g. T_3 and T_4). Around 10% of T_4 is converted to T_3 in the follicular cell cytoplasm by deiodinase enzymes. Ninety per cent of thyroid hormones are secreted in the form of T_4 with the remainder as T_3. Eighty per cent of the T_4 is converted to the more active T_3 (under the stimulation of TSH) in the liver and kidney or to reverse T_3 (rT_3) that has little or no biological activity. MIT and DIT are also released, but they are deiodinated by iodotyrosine dehalogenase to recycle iodine.

Iodine metabolism

Iodine is acquired from the diet mainly from iodized salt, meat and vegetables. About 150 mg of iodine is needed per day, though only a fraction of this is absorbed. The thyroid gland cells are the only cells that can actively absorb and utilize plasma iodine; a considerable quantity of iodine is stored in the

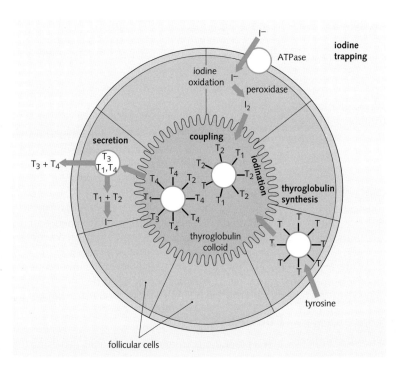

Fig. 3.6 Steps in the synthesis and secretion of T_3 and T_4. (T_3, tri-iodothyronine; T_4, thyroxine.)

thyroid as preformed thyroid hormones. Iodine is returned to the plasma by the breakdown of these thyroid hormones. Iodine is excreted mainly via the kidneys.

> Thiacarbimide drugs, such as carbimazole, used in the treatment of hyperthyroidism, inhibit thyroid peroxidase. This inhibition results in decreased oxidation of iodide, decreased iodination of iodides and ultimately reduced thyroid hormone production.

Regulation

Thyroid activity is controlled by the hypothalamus and anterior pituitary. Hypothalamic thyrotrophin-releasing hormone (TRH) is released into the hypophyseal portal blood and this stimulates the release of thyroid-stimulating hormone (TSH or thyrotrophin) from the anterior pituitary gland. This happens in response to several things, including low thyroid hormone levels, cold, pregnancy, etc. TSH acts on extracellular receptors on the surface of thyroid follicle cells. Cyclic AMP (cAMP) is formed and this stimulates five of the stages of synthesis and secretion:

- Iodine uptake
- Thyroglobulin synthesis
- Iodination

- Coupling
- Pinocytosis for secretion.

As a result, T_3 and T_4 are synthesized and secreted more rapidly. TSH also has long-term actions on the thyroid gland by increasing its size and vascularity to improve hormone synthesis.

A number of factors affect thyroid hormone release. Three main factors stimulate secretion:

- Long-term exposure to cold temperatures acting on the anterior pituitary
- Oestrogens acting on the anterior pituitary
- Adrenaline (epinephrine) acting directly on the thyroid gland.

A negative feedback loop exists to partly maintain temperature homeostasis and circulating levels of T_3 and T_4. TSH secretion is inhibited by raised serum levels of thyroid hormones, as well as somatostatin, glucocorticoids and chronic illness. The regulatory effect comes from thyroid hormones acting on the pituitary receptors to TRH as opposed to reducing TRH secretion from the hypothalamus. High levels of iodine also suppress secretion of thyroid hormones.

Transport of thyroid hormones

Most of the thyroid hormones in the blood are bound to plasma proteins produced within the liver, which allows them to circulate without being broken down by enzymes. The transport is also necessary as T_3 and T_4

are lipophilic molecules, meaning that they will not readily dissolve in the blood.

- 70% are bound to thyroid-binding globulin (TBG)
- 30% are bound to albumin.

Only a fraction of the circulating thyroid hormones (0.1% of T_4 and 1% of T_3) is unbound/free and biologically active. Bound hormone cannot diffuse into the body's cells.

Actions

Thyroid hormones are responsible in part for the expression of genes in target cells. They are mediated by the same receptors as all steroid hormones (Chapter 1); however, thyroid hormone receptors are found in the nucleus, not the cytoplasm. Fig. 3.7 shows some of the differences between T_3 and T_4. T_4 is a relatively inactive, stable molecule that can be thought of as a prohormone and provides a reservoir for the more active T_3. T_3 is found in a higher percentage of active hormone than T_4 and has a greater effect on receptors. The benefit to the production of two hormones is that T_4 can maintain a background level of activity whilst T_3 levels can adapt quickly to changing environments.

Peripheral tissues and organs, e.g. the liver, spleen and kidneys, have the ability to regulate local T_3 levels

by increasing or decreasing T_3 synthesis. T_4 is converted to T_3 by deiodination, i.e. removal of one iodine atom catalysed by deiodinase enzymes. Two main forms of this enzyme have been found:

- Type 1 – found on the cell surface in most tissues. It raises local T_3.
- Type 2 – intracellular enzymes that raise cellular T_3 in the central nervous system (CNS) and pituitary gland.

A further deiodinase enzyme can remove a different iodine molecule from T_4 to form reverse T_3 (rT_3). This is an inactive molecule that binds to the receptor sites in the nucleus and blocks the actions of T_3. Excess rT_3 can lead to a condition called *reverse T_3 syndrome*. RT_3 is produced in larger quantities when energy stores are low or in periods of illness, so as to conserve energy.

In general, T_3 promotes energy production in every cell in the body by increasing the size and number of mitochondria. This causes heat production and maintains metabolism. Fig. 3.8 shows the intracellular actions of T_3.

Feedback

T_3 receptors are also found in the pituitary gland and the hypothalamus, where they inhibit transcription of the gene for TRH prohormone and the release of TSH, respectively. Excess T_3 inhibits TSH release while a deficiency of T_3 stimulates TSH release. This feedback mechanism helps maintain T_3 levels, and therefore stabilizes metabolic rate.

Fig. 3.7 Comparison of T_3 and T_4

	T_3	T_4
Proportion of secreted thyroid hormone	10%	90%
Percentage free in plasma	1%	0.1%
Relative activity	10	1
Half-life (days)	1	7

DISORDERS OF THE THYROID GLAND

The thyroid gland is prone to a number of diseases that can alter its function and structure. These diseases frequently have wide-ranging systemic effects because

Fig. 3.8 Intracellular and physiological actions of T_3

Site of action	Intracellular effects	Physiological results
Cell membrane	Stimulates the Na+/K+ATPase pump	Increased demand for metabolites, e.g. glucose
Mitochondria	Stimulates growth, replication and activity; basal metabolic rate is raised	Increased heat production, oxygen demand, heart rate and stroke volume
Nucleus	Increases expression of enzymes necessary for energy production	Lipolysis, glycolysis and gluconeogenesis increased to raise blood metabolite levels and cellular metabolite use
Neonatal cells	Essential for cell division and maturation	Essential for normal development of CNS and skeleton

thyroid hormones regulate the metabolism of almost every cell in the body. The main categories of disease are:

- Hyperthyroidism – excess of thyroid hormone production
- Hypothyroidism – deficiency of thyroid hormone production
- Goitre formation
- Adenoma (benign growths) of the thyroid
- Carcinoma.

Clinical examination and findings of thyroid disorders are discussed later in the chapter.

Hyperthyroidism

This can be defined as *'overactivity of the thyroid gland, either due to a tumour, overgrowth of the gland, or Graves' disease'* that can lead to an excess of thyroid hormone secretion. When this becomes symptomatic, it causes a condition known as thyrotoxicosis. This is a common endocrine disorder affecting two in 100 women and two in 1000 men and can develop at any age. Hyperthyroidism can present in a number of ways, with some variation depending on the underlying cause. These are shown in Fig. 3.9.

The classic presentation is usually a gradual weight loss despite increased appetite (NB there as a paradoxical weight gain in 10–30% of cases).

An acute exacerbation of symptoms can be called a few names that are all very similar, including thyroid storm or thyrotoxic storm. This is commonly precipitated by recent thyroid surgery (damaged follicles releasing their contents), infection, myocardial infarctions, etc., and is considered to be a medical emergency requiring immediate treatment by an experienced endocrinologist. The main causes of hyperthyroidism are:

- Graves' disease – an autoimmune disease
- Toxic mulitnodular goitre – nodules develop that secrete thyroid hormones, most commonly seen in elderly patients and in populations where iodine intake is too low.
- Toxic adenoma – a benign growth that secretes T_3 and T_4.

Additional (and rarer) causes include subacute (de Quervain's) thyroiditis, ectopic thyroid tissue, drugs, e.g. amiodarone or thyroxine, overdose.

Diagnosis

Thyroid function tests are the main method of diagnosis. Serum TSH, free T_3 and free T_4 are measured by radioimmunoassay (RIA). Elevated T_3 and T_4 levels indicate hyperthyroidism is present. Raised TSH suggests the fault lies in or above the pituitary gland, whereas low TSH points to a thyroid organ disorder.

Fig. 3.9 Symptoms and signs of thyrotoxicosis (hyperthyroidism). The features in italic are only found in Graves' disease.

Hair	loss
Brain	emotional lability
	fatigue
	anxiety
	restlessness
Eyes	*exophtalmos*
	lid retraction
	lid lag
	predisposes to keratitis
Neck	goitre
Heart	palpations
	tachycardia (rapid pulse)
	atrial fibrillation
Muscles	Proximal myopathy (in upper arms and legs)
Bowel	diarrhoea
	increased appetite
Hands	tremor
	warmth
	sweating
Uterus	menorrhagia
	infertility
	reduced libido
Bones	oesteoporosis
Reflexes	increased
Skin and adipose tissue	increased sweating
	heat intolerance
	weight loss
	pretibial myxoedema

Other tests include:

- Autoantibody screening, e.g. Graves' disease
- Radioisotope scanning to show the size of the thyroid gland and any abnormal 'hot' areas such as a toxic adenoma
- ECG to check for sinus tachycardia or atrial fibrillation (as a result of excess thyroid hormones).

Treatment

Treatment varies depending on the cause of the hyperthyroidism and requires specialist monitoring and control in infancy and pregnancy. The main treatments, however, can be divided into three methods:

1. Drug therapy: β-blockers for rapid symptomatic control, e.g. palpitations, anxiety.

   Carbimazole inhibits the peroxidase reactions of T_3 and T_4 synthesis but can take around a month to have a marked effect. Some physicians use a block–replace method, i.e. treat with carbimazole and thyroxine simultaneously to avoid risk of iatrogenic hypothyroidism.

2. Radioiodine (^{131}I): ^{131}I is only absorbed by the thyroid tissue, killing the cells and reducing thyroid hormone synthesis. The response is slow and carbimazole may still be required.

3. Partial thyroidectomy: The thyroid gland is removed surgically leaving some tissue and the parathyroid glands.

Both radioiodine and partial thyroidectomy run the risk of long-term hypothyroidism as the remaining thyroid tissue may not be sufficient to meet the body's demands, especially with increasing age. Their treatment is described under hypothyroidism.

Graves' disease

Graves' disease is an autoimmune disease, in which autoantibodies against the TSH receptors are produced. These antibodies stimulate the TSH receptors and lead to an excess production of thyroid hormones. Autoantibodies to thyroglobulin and to the thyroid hormones may also be produced. Graves' disease is the most common cause of hyperthyroidism and thyrotoxicosis; and is especially common in middle-aged women ($♀:♂$, 8:1). There is a genetic association with the human leucocyte antigen (HLA).

The disease itself follows either a relapsing–remitting course or one with fluctuating severity. Graves' can lead to hypothyroidism in some rare cases.

Classically, Graves' disease presents with a 'staring' appearance (exophthalmos), a goitre (with bruit) and swollen legs (pretibial myxoedema).

Graves' ophthalmopathy is caused by lymphocytic infiltration of the periorbital tissues and activation of fibroblasts to secrete osmotically active hyaluronic acid. This increases the pressure and pushes the eye forward, resulting in proptosis. This pressure change also causes muscle fibrosis and diplopia due to weakening of the extraocular muscles. Corneal ulcers are also important to be aware of and inflammation can cause optic nerve compression. The eye disease may precede the onset of thyroid dysfunction, and does not respond to correction of thyroid status. Treatment involves radiotherapy and surgery.

Graves' disease is diagnosed by detection of autoantibodies along with low TSH and raised T_4 and/or T_3.

The thyroid autoantibodies, thyroglobulin antibody (TgAb) and thyroid peroxidase (TPO) antibody, are present in both Graves' disease and Hashimoto's thyroiditis. However, thyroid receptor antibody (TRAb) or thyroid-stimulating hormone receptor (TSH-R) antibodies are specific to Graves' disease. The treatment is consistent with other causes of hyperthyroidism, but radioactive iodine and surgery are especially likely to cause hypothyroidism.

Thyroid hormone resistance syndrome

This is a rare condition that occurs due to a mutation in one of the thyroid receptor genes. In most cases the raised levels of T_3 and T_4 compensate for the resistance, but 'generalized resistance' can present with congenital hypothyroidism.

Hypothyroidism

Hypothyroidism is defined as an underactive thyroid gland leading to deficient thyroid hormones (T_3 and T_4). When this becomes symptomatic, it is called myxoedema. It is slightly less common than hyperthyroidism, affecting 1/100 females and 1/500 males. The symptoms and signs of myxoedema are illustrated in Fig. 3.10. Presentation is even more gradual than hyperthyroidism, many symptoms frequently being ignored.

Thyroid hormones are essential between birth and puberty for the normal development of the CNS. Deficiency can cause irreversible mental retardation called cretinism. TSH levels are checked in all newborns for this relatively common abnormality; the levels will be raised if the thyroid gland is not functioning correctly.

Diagnosis

Hypothyroidism is not investigated as thoroughly as hyperthyroidism, since treatment does not vary. Free T_3 and T_4 levels are low, whereas TSH levels are usually raised. If TSH is low then a lesion of the hypothalamus or pituitary is likely. Autoantibodies can be detected in Hashimoto's thyroiditis.

Treatment

All hypothyroidism is treated with thyroxine (T_4) administered as an oral tablet in varying doses. The dose is increased over several months, with regular monitoring of TSH levels until they are within the normal boundaries. This process is slow, since it takes 4 weeks for TSH levels to reflect an increased dose due to the long half-life of thyroxine. Thyroxine therapy is usually maintained for life.

Fig. 3.10 Symptoms and signs of myxoedema (hypothyroidism). The main features are shown in bold.	
Hair	**coarse and thin hair**
	loss of outer third of eyebrows
Brain	**mental slowing**
	apathy
	tiredness
	psychosis
Face	myxoedemic features, ie. **pale puffy face**, coarse features
	deafness
Throat	hoarse voice
Neck	goitre
Heart	brachycardia (slow pulse)
Muscles	slowing of activity
	muscle weakness in upper arms and legs (proximal myopathy)
Bowel	constipation
Hands	cold hands
	carpel tunnel syndrome
Reflexes	slow relaxing
Skin and adipose tissue	**weight gain/obesity**
	intolerance to cold
	decreased sweating
	chronic oedema (caused by increased capillary escape of albumin)
	cold, dry skin

Over-treatment of hyperthyroidism

Radioactive ablation and surgical removal of the thyroid gland initially cure hyperthyroidism, but with time, the remaining thyroid tissue is often insufficient. Hypothyroidism can develop and lifelong thyroxine treatment is required.

Many drugs can also cause reversible hypothyroidism including lithium, amiodarone and excess iodine.

Hashimoto's thyroiditis

When the thyroid gland is inflamed, the disease is called thyroiditis. This can be caused by autoimmune or viral processes. Hashimoto's thyroiditis is a destructive autoimmune disease that is especially common in middle-aged women. It is mediated by autoantibodies against rough endoplasmic reticulum (microsomal antibodies) or thyroglobulin. The presence of these antibodies can

be tested to confirm the diagnosis. The thyroid gland is infiltrated by lymphocytes that cause the gland to enlarge, forming a goitre.

The initial destruction of the thyroid gland can release the thyroglobulin colloid causing temporary hyperthyroidism. The patients usually progress to a euthyroid (normal) state and finally develop progressive hypothyroidism.

De Quervain's (subacute) thyroiditis

De Quervain's thyroiditis is inflammation of the thyroid gland caused by a virus. It is common in young or middle-aged women, in whom it causes a tender swollen gland along with a febrile illness. The inflammation causes an initial increase in thyroid hormone release followed by destroying the follicles, which causes hypothyroidism and leakage of the thyroglobulin colloid. An immune reaction against this colloid causes the formation of granulomas, so this disease is also called granulomatous thyroiditis.

Primary atrophic hypothyroidism

Spontaneous or primary atrophic hypothyroidism is a disease resulting in hypothyroidism in the elderly. The biochemical profile may include the presence of TSH-R-blocking autoantibodies, but in this condition the thyroid fibroses and shrinks so that there is no goitre. It is suspected that this disease is the end-stage of many thyroid diseases, including Hashimoto's and de Quervain's thyroiditis.

Dyshormonogenesis

This is an inherited defect in the synthesis of thyroid hormones, and can present with hypothyroidism and goitre.

Iodine deficiency

Iodine deficiency was once a common cause of goitre in regions where the soil lacked iodine (e.g. Derbyshire, England), but nowadays iodine is added to salt to prevent this. Deficient iodine means that thyroid hormones cannot be synthesized, with a resultant rise in TSH levels. TSH causes thyroid enlargement by stimulating follicle growth and the development of new blood vessels, so the thyroid gland enlarges.

Goitres

A goitre is a swelling in the neck caused by an enlarged thyroid gland. It is a common finding, and it is usually asymptomatic; however, large goitres can compress the oesophagus and trachea. If a goitre is associated with hyperthyroidism it is described as 'toxic'. Non-toxic goitres secrete normal or reduced levels of thyroid hormones. Non-toxic goitres are usually the result of excessive TSH stimulation in the presence of hypothyroidism. Goitres are treated by correcting the underlying pathology or by surgical removal for cosmetic reasons or to prevent compression of surrounding structures.

Iodine deficiency

The goitre formed by this process is diffusely enlarged and smooth. It is sometimes called an endemic goitre because it occurred in certain regions.

Graves' disease

The constant stimulation of TSH receptors in Graves' disease causes a goitre in a similar manner to iodine deficiency with similar characteristics. The gland becomes very vascular, to the extent that a bruit can be heard using a stethoscope.

Puberty and pregnancy

Higher levels of thyroid hormones are required in puberty and pregnancy so the thyroid gland often enlarges to meet the increased demand. This enlargement is a physiological response, not a pathological process. The goitre regresses once the demand lessens.

Multinodular goitre

Many elderly people have an enlarged thyroid that contains many nodules of varying sizes. These nodules are formed from hyperplasia (increased number) of thyroid cells. The excess cells sometimes cause excess thyroid hormone production, i.e. hyperthyroidism. The disease is then called toxic multinodular goitre.

Thyroiditis

Inflammation of the thyroid gland can cause swelling, and infiltration by lymphocytes can also cause enlargement. The goitre formed is usually slightly nodular, but it may be tender if the inflammation is acute.

Thyroid gland neoplasia

Thyroid lumps are common and usually benign; however, they must be investigated. Solitary thyroid lumps are found in 5% of women and it is very difficult to distinguish between benign (80%) and malignant (20%) on clinical grounds. A fine-needle aspiration should be performed along with thyroid function tests. Aspiration alone will not distinguish a follicular adenoma from a follicular carcinoma but low TSH suggests the former as malignant nodules are not usually hyperfunctioning.

Causes of solitary thyroid lumps include:

- Thyroid cysts
- Nodule of multinodular goitre
- Follicular adenoma
- Malignancy.

Five separate forms of cancer can arise in the thyroid gland, but three of these are derived from the follicle cells. These tumours are summarized in Fig. 3.11.

Medullary carcinomas of the parafollicular cells often secrete ectopic hormones, including:

- Calcitonin – usually asymptomatic
- Adrenocorticotrophic hormone (ACTH) – Cushing's syndrome
- 5-hydroxytryptamine (5-HT; serotonin) – carcinoid syndrome.

The molecular biology of thyroid cancer

A great deal has been learnt about the molecular biology of thyroid cancer. Fifty per cent of papillary thyroid cancers have a translocation that causes

Fig. 3.11 Characteristics of the five primary thyroid gland malignancies				
Type	Cell type	Age group	Route of metastasis	Prognosis
Papillary	Follicle cells	All	Cervical lymphatics	Excellent
Follicular	Follicle cells	Middle-aged	Blood to bone, lung and brain	Good
Medullary	Parafollicular cells	Middle-aged and elderly	Cervical lymphatics	Variable but usually good
Malignant lymphoma	Lymphatics	Elderly	Local invasion	Poor
Anaplastic	Follicle cells	Elderly	Local invasion	Very poor

constitutive activation of the *RET* proto-oncogene. *RET* is a transmembrane receptor with tyrosine kinase activity, which when active can drive oncogenesis (the development of neoplasia). In follicular thyroid cancer (FTC), 40% of cases have an activating point mutation of the *RAS* proto-oncogene; 60% of FTCs were shown to produce an abnormal 'fusion protein' (PAX-8/PPARγ), which is the result of two gene fragments coming together by translocation and producing a single gene product. Medullary thyroid cancer often occurs as part of the multiple endocrine neoplasia syndrome and as such is often associated with *RET* mutations. The more aggressive form, anaplastic thyroid cancer, is often associated with a *p53* mutation. This new knowledge of the events driving thyroid neoplastic transformation has opened up novel avenues for therapy.

Medical emergencies of the thyroid

Occasionally, thyroid disorders present as an emergency.

A thyrotoxic crisis/ thyroid storm is an acute severe attack of hyperthyroidism, usually precipitated by thyroid surgery, infection, trauma and radioiodine therapy. Signs and symptoms include pyrexia, confusion, diarrhoea, vomiting, coma and life-threatening arrhythmias. The diagnosis can be confirmed using a technetium scan, but this should come second to urgent treatment. Treatment is with beta-blockers and antithyroid therapy, with additional treatments to treat the underlying cause, e.g. antibiotics for infection.

Myxoedema coma is another emergency, associated with hypothyroidism, precipitated by infection, stroke, myocardial infarction and trauma. A history of treatment for hyperthyroidism, e.g. surgery or radioiodine therapy, is common. Signs and symptoms include hypothermia, hyporeflexia, hypoglycaemia, bradycardia, coma and seizures.

Examination of the thyroid

Signs of thyroid disease are elucidated by examining the energetic state of the patient. The main components of any examination are inspection, palpation, percussion and auscultation.

Inspection

The patient will look different depending on the problem with the thyroid. The general signs and symptoms for hyperthyroidism are shown in Fig. 3.9 and hypothyroidism in Fig. 3.10.

Closer inspection may reveal further pathology (Figs 3.12 and 3.13).

Fig 3.12 Common findings in hyperthyroidism

Face	Lid lag – slow descent of the upper eye lid, lags behind the eyeball movement. Lid retraction – at rest, the superior limbus of the iris and possibly even some of the sclera (white of the eye) is visible. Exophthalmos – the eye bulges beyond the socket and it is possible to see the whole iris and sometimes even sclera surrounding its circumference
Skin	Flushed, red skin and excessive sweating
Hands	Warm and moist palms, fine tremor, clubbing (soft tissue swelling at the nail base), onycholysis (separation of the nail from the bed) and whiting of the nail tip
Pulse	Tachycardia (pulse > 100 bpm), irregular rhythm (signifies cardiac arrhythmia, seen in thyrotoxicosis)
Neck	Goitre
Limbs	Pretibial myxoedema (thickened skin over the tibia, with elevated dermal nodules and plaques; only seen in Graves' disease), proximal wasting (seen in the biceps and quadriceps), exaggerated reflexes

Fig 3.13 Common findings in hypothyroidism

Face	Puffy face, coarse features, coarse dry hair, loss of eyebrows, hoarse voice, swollen tongue. In infants, a broad, flat face, widely spaced eyes and a protruding tongue may be seen (cretinism)
Skin	Cold and dry
Hands	Palms are cold and dry
Pulse	Bradycardia (pulse < 60 bpm)
Neck	Goitre
Limbs	Proximal muscle wasting (seen in the biceps and quadriceps)

Examination of the neck, eyes and legs is very important for the thyroid. Anterior and lateral inspection of the neck can reveal thyroid masses. Patients are asked to swallow some water and thyroid masses will move with the trachea. Palpation of the thyroid isthmus and lobes looks for any displacement, enlargement and/or nodules. The thyroid can also be palpated during swallowing. A full examination would include palpation of regional lymph nodes.

Percussion is only used to detect any enlargement of the thyroid inferiorly to behind the sternum. Percussion of the sternum is dull in the presence of a retrosternal mass.

Auscultation is of the arteries in the neck to detect any bruits (turbulent blood flow) due to increased vascularity.

Investigations and imaging of the thyroid

Investigation of thyroid function overlaps with pituitary testing as thyroid disorders can be secondary to pituitary problems. One method for investigating the thyroid is hormone assays.

Hormone assays

If abnormalities of thyroid function are suspected then plasma levels of TSH, T_4 and T_3 should be measured. Both thyroid hormones should be measured because variations in thyroxine-binding globulin (TBG) levels can give inaccurate results. Further investigations are often not needed:

- Low levels of T_4 and T_3 – hypothyroidism
- High levels of T_4 and T_3 – hyperthyroidism.

TSH is measured with T_4 and T_3 to locate the lesion. In hypothyroidism a low TSH suggests a pituitary/hypothalamus lesion while a high TSH suggests a thyroid gland problem. In hyperthyroidism, TSH will almost always be low as pituitary and hypothalamic lesions causing high TSH are rare.

TSH is also measured to guide thyroxine treatment of thyroid disorders. The correct dose of thyroxine or carbimazole is being administered when TSH levels return to normal.

Thyrotrophin-releasing hormone stimulation test

This stimulation test is used if TSH deficiency due to pituitary lesion is suspected. Hypothalamic TRH is administered intravenously and plasma TSH levels are measured before and after to assess pituitary response.

Thyroid autoantibody assay

ELISA (enzyme-linked immunosorbent assay) can also be used to detect thyroid autoantibodies caused by the common autoimmune thyroid diseases:

- Thyroid receptor antibodies (TRAb) suggest Graves' disease
- Anti-thyroid peroxidase (anti-TPO) and anti-thyroglobulin (anti-TgAb) antibodies suggest Hashimoto's thyroiditis.

Management of thyroid nodules varies between hospitals. Findings of irregular firm nodules, lymph node involvement or tethering to surrounding structures on clinical examination are suggestive of malignancy. Ultrasound and thyroid biochemistry are usually used as the first-line investigations, Malignancy is more commonly associated with euthyroidism or hypothyroidism and hypo-echoic lesions on ultrasound. Isotope scans can reveal 'hot' (functioning – and less likely to be malignant) and 'cold' (non-functioning) nodules. If thyroid biochemistry is within the normal range and nodules are 'cold', fine-needle aspiration biopsy (FNAC) can be performed as the most sensitive and specific test for confirming a diagnosis of malignancy.

The adrenal glands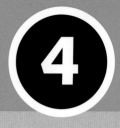

By the end of this chapter you should be able to:
- Explain the structure and development of the adrenal glands
- Describe the synthesis of adrenal hormones
- Understand the regulation and physiological effects of adrenal hormones
- Discuss the major disorders associated with adrenal function.

The two adrenal glands are incredibly important because the hormones they secrete enable the body to respond to the stresses of life, both emotional and physical.

The adrenal glands are located on the superior pole of each kidney. During embryonic development the adrenal gland forms two functionally distinct regions, each with a different embryological origin. The outer, larger region is called the adrenal cortex and the inner, much smaller, adrenal medulla.

The **adrenal cortex** is controlled by the pituitary gland, responding to a hormone called adrenocorticotrophic hormone (ACTH). The cells of the cortex secrete three steroid hormones and each has a distinctly different function from the others.

- Glucocorticoids – produced in response to stress
- Mineralocorticoids – regulate blood volume
- Androgens – control sexual development.

The **adrenal medulla** is composed of sympathetic nerve cells, though the cells here have no axons. It has the same embryonic origin as sympathetic nerves and is considered a modified sympathetic ganglion of the autonomic nervous system (ANS). The cells of the medulla are under the direct control of the sympathetic nervous system, which causes it to secrete two amino acid hormones. These act to enhance the effects the sympathetic division of the ANS has on the rest of the body during stress.

- Adrenaline (epinephrine)
- Noradrenaline (norepinephrine).

The most important hormones produced by the adrenal glands are glucocorticoids, such as cortisol. This hormone has the very important function in normal life as it can protect humans from stress-induced hypotension, shock and death. Synthetic glucocorticoids are known as 'steroids' or 'corticosteroids' and are commonly used in the treatment of acute inflammatory diseases. The mechanism that controls the release of these hormones is a negative-feedback system known as the hypothalamic–pituitary–adrenal (HPA) axis (Fig 4.1).

An excess of glucocorticoid causes Cushing's syndrome and a deficiency causes Addison's disease.

Another important hormone to note is adrenaline, which is used as an emergency treatment in situations such as anaphylactic shock or cardiac arrest.

ANATOMY

There are two adrenal glands (also called suprarenal glands in America), associated with the superior aspect of each kidney. However, each adrenal gland has a different shape and relation to the other. As previously mentioned the glands have an inner and outer region, each with its own individual controls and secretions, so they can be thought of as a gland within a gland. The glands are retroperitoneal, covered in perinephric fat and enclosed in renal fascia; however, there is a thin septum which separates each gland from its associated kidney.

Right adrenal gland

The right gland is shaped like a pyramid and is located posterior to the right lobe of the liver. The inferior vena cava and the right crus of the diaphragm lie medial and lateral, respectively, to the adrenal gland.

Left adrenal gland

The left gland is the larger of the pair and is crescent-shaped. Anterior to the gland is part of the pancreas, stomach and occasionally the spleen. The left crus of the diaphragm lies laterally. The diaphragm also lies posterior to both adrenal glands (Fig 4.2).

By comparison, the venous drainage is much simpler than the arterial supply. The **right adrenal vein** is short and immediately enters the inferior vena cava, whereas the **left adrenal gland** travels inferior to enter the left renal vein.

The outer cortex receives no significant innervations; instead it is regulated by ACTH from the pituitary gland and other bloodborne factors.

The medulla is innervated directly by the splanchnic nerves, which arise from the thoracic spinal cord and do not synapse before reaching the adrenal medulla. The nerves are therefore preganglionic sympathetic nerves that release acetylcholine, while all other tissues receive postganglionic sympathetic innervations. The cause of this relationship is apparent from their development (see below).

Lymphatic drainage of the adrenal glands is through the para-aortic nodes.

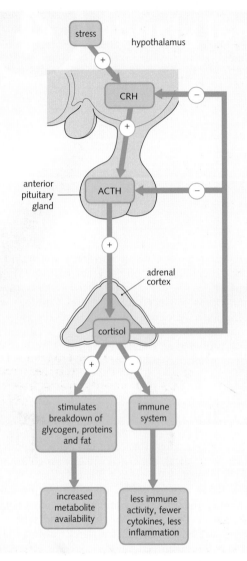

Fig. 4.1 Hormonal regulation of cortisol. (ACTH, adrenocorticotrophic hormone; CRH, corticotrophin-releasing hormone.)

Blood supply, nerves and lymphatics

The blood supply to the adrenal glands is massive and comes from three main sources:

- **Superior suprarenal arteries** – multiple branches from the inferior phrenic arteries as they pass upward from the abdominal aorta
- **Middle suprarenal artery** – branches off directly from the abdominal aorta
- **Inferior suprarenal arteries** – inferior branches from the renal arteries ascend to supply the glands.

DEVELOPMENT

Adrenal cortex

The adrenal cortex develops from mesodermal cells that lie adjacent to the urogenital ridge. The fetal zone of the cortex develops first. Later, more mesodermal cells surround the fetal cortex to form the permanent cortex found in adults. At birth, the permanent cortex has two layers, while a third (the zona reticularis) develops by the third year of life. At around this time the fetal cortex regresses until only the developed medulla and permanent cortex are left.

The zona reticularis matures around the age of 8 years old and begins to secrete weak androgens. This is called adrenarche and is discussed later.

Adrenal medulla

The adrenal medulla is derived from ectodermal neural crest cells of the embryo. They form part of the amine precursor uptake and decarboxylation (APUD) system. These cells contribute to many diverse structures, including all the noradrenaline-secreting postganglionic neurons in the sympathetic nervous system. The secretory cells in the adrenal medulla secrete either adrenaline or noradrenaline, and they are essentially highly specialized neurons (Fig. 4.3). The medullary precursor cells also form paraganglia in the organ of Zuckerkandl located around the origin of the inferior mesenteric artery and the aortic bifurcation, which act as accessory medullary tissue and are a common site of extra-adrenal catecholamine-secreting tumours.

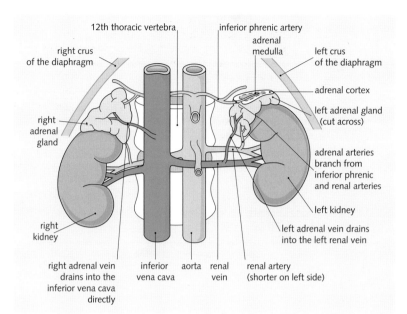

Fig. 4.2 Location and blood supply of the adrenal glands.

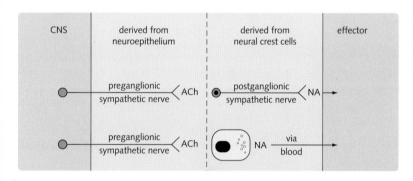

Fig. 4.3 Comparison between the adrenal medulla and the sympathetic nervous system (ACh, acetylcholine; CNS, central nervous system; NA, noradrenaline).

MICROSTRUCTURE

Adrenal cortex

The adult adrenal cortex makes up about 90% of the adrenal gland by weight. It is functionally and anatomically divided into three layers, which secrete the following groups of steroid hormone (Figs 4.4 and 4.5):

- Outer zona glomerulosa secretes mineralocorticoids
- Middle zona fasciculata secretes glucocorticoids
- Inner zona reticularis secretes androgens and glucocorticoids.

These hormone groups will be explained later in this chapter.

The cells of the zona fasciculata and zona reticularis are arranged in columns around blood sinusoids.

The blood in these sinusoids passes directly into the adrenal medulla.

Adrenal medulla

The adrenal medulla comprises two types of neuroendocrine cell:

- Noradrenaline-secreting cells (20%)
- Adrenaline-secreting cells (80%).

Both types contain neuroendocrine granules that store the hormone. In older textbooks, these cells are called chromaffin cells because they turn a dark-brown colour if exposed to oxygen after fixation in chrome salts. The cells are arranged around blood sinusoids.

Medullary cells require the steroid cortisol to convert noradrenaline to adrenaline. Cortisol is produced in the cortex, and it travels in the cortical capillaries to the medulla. Separate medullary arteries supply oxygenated blood directly.

Fig. 4.4 Microstructure of the adrenal gland and the major hormones secreted in each region

Region	Name	Cell structure	Hormones synthesized
Outer cortex	Zona glomerulosa	Cells arranged in clumps (Latin, glomerulus: little ball)	Mineralocorticoids (mainly aldosterone)
Middle cortex	Zona fasciculata	Cells arranged in cords alongside blood sinusoids; (Latin, fasciculus: bundle)	Glucocorticoids (mainly cortisol)
Inner cortex	Zona reticularis	Network of smaller cells (Latin, reticularis: network)	Glucocorticoids and androgens (DHEA)
Centre of gland	Adrenal medulla	Loose network of neurosecretory cells surrounded by blood sinusoids	Catecholamines (adrenaline and noradrenaline)

DHEA, dehydroepiandrosterone.

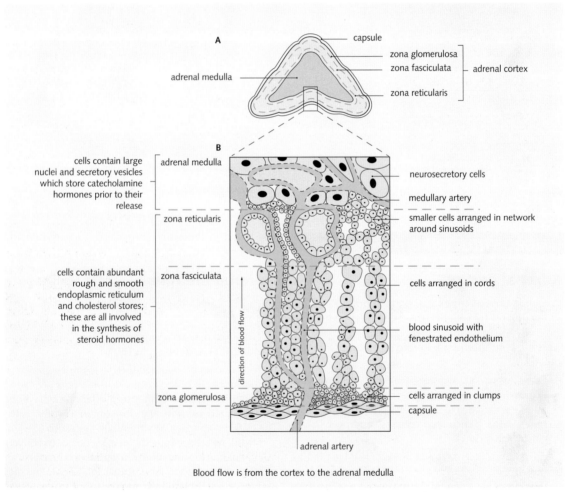

Blood flow is from the cortex to the adrenal medulla

Fig. 4.5 Microstructure of a cross-section through the adrenal glands showing the cell types and regions.

HORMONES OF THE ADRENAL CORTEX

The adrenal cortex secretes three groups of steroid hormones:

- Mineralocorticoids, e.g. aldosterone, deoxycortisone
- Glucocorticoids, e.g. cortisol
- Androgens, e.g. dehydroepiandrosterone (DHEA).

Steroid hormones are synthesized from cholesterol. Steroid hormones are small lipid-soluble molecules that cross membranes readily. Inside cells, they act on intracellular receptors to regulate gene expression. The synthesis and mechanism of action of steroid hormones are discussed in more detail in Chapter 1.

MINERALOCORTICOIDS AND ALDOSTERONE

Regulation of aldosterone

Mineralocorticoids help to regulate the electronic balance of plasma; their name is derived from this action on the body's minerals. Aldosterone is the main mineralcorticoid secreted by the zona glomerulosa. Aldosterone release is stimulated by:

- Angiotensin II
- High plasma potassium
- ACTH.

Angiotensin II is released in response to low blood volume as part of the renin–angiotensin system (see Chapter 7 and Fig. 4.6). ACTH from the anterior pituitary gland is less important as a regulator, so pituitary failure does not severely impair aldosterone secretion. An excess of aldosterone due to an adrenal adenoma is called Conn's disease.

Actions of aldosterone

Aldosterone acts mainly on the distal convoluted tubule (DCT) and the collecting duct of the kidney. It causes reabsorption of sodium ions in exchange for potassium and hydrogen ions. Water is also reabsorbed and blood volume is increased. Other hormones are involved in this mechanism and they are discussed in more detail in Chapter 7 on fluid balance.

Intracellular actions of aldosterone

To cause these physiological effects, aldosterone acts on the nucleus via an intracellular receptor. Only cells that express this receptor can respond to aldosterone.

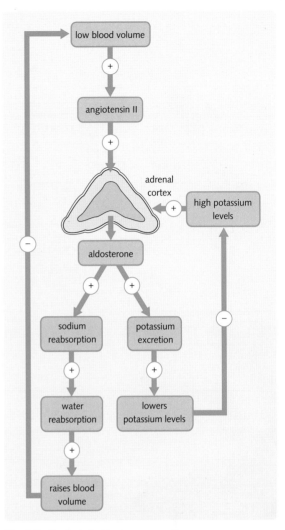

Fig. 4.6 Control of aldosterone secretion.

Aldosterone up-regulates the expression of four genes in the cells of the DCT and collecting duct. The actions of the gene products (proteins) are described in Fig. 4.7.

Aldosterone circulates in the plasma with 60% bound to albumin and 40% free, and therefore active. The high proportion of free hormone causes aldosterone to be rapidly degraded by the liver, giving a short half-life of about 15 minutes.

GLUCOCORTICOIDS AND CORTISOL

Glucocorticoids regulate the metabolism of carbohydrate, protein and, to a lesser extent, fat. Glucocorticoids also have potent anti-inflammatory and immunosuppressive effects. The major glucocorticoid in humans is

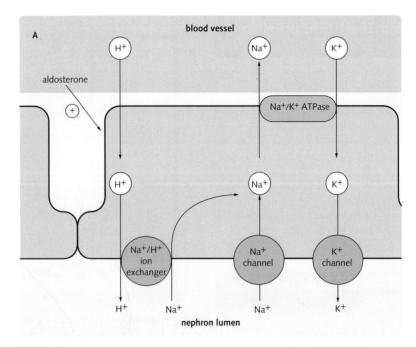

Fig. 4.7B Effects of proteins induced by aldosterone in the nephron

Protein	Location	Action	Physiological response
Na⁺/K⁺ ATPase	Cell membrane on the side of the blood supply	Active pump that increases cell potassium and lowers cell sodium levels	Creates an ion gradient that drives the other proteins
Na⁺ channel	Cell membrane on the side of the nephron	Reabsorbs sodium from the nephron lumen	Increases plasma sodium and water to increase blood volume
K⁺ channel	Cell membrane on the side of the nephron	Excretes potassium into the nephron lumen	Decreases plasma potassium
Na⁺/H⁺ ion exchanger	Cell membrane on the side of the nephron	Reabsorbs sodium in exchange for hydrogen ions	Makes the plasma more alkaline

Fig. 4.7 Intracellular and physiological actions of aldosterone in the nephron. Aldosterone acts to increase the levels of the four proteins shown (A) causing the physiological responses (B).

cortisol. Cortisol also plays an important part in metabolic adaptation in response to stressful stimuli.

During fasting, glucocorticoids act to maintain plasma glucose levels.

Regulation of cortisol

Corticotrophin-releasing hormone (CRH) is secreted by the hypothalamus and stimulates the anterior pituitary to produce pro-opiomelanocortin (POMC), which is converted to ACTH and leads to increased ACTH release. ACTH, in turn, acts on G-protein-coupled receptors on the wall of the adrenal cells to stimulate steroidogenesis. Vasopressin can increase the ability of CRH to cause ACTH release. Cortisol has a negative feedback effect on the hypothalamus (inhibits CRH transcription) and anterior pituitary gland (inhibits POMC transcription) to inhibit CRH and ACTH release.

Cortisol release displays a circadian rhythm, i.e. the rate of secretion changes through a 24-hour period (Fig. 4.8). The highest levels of cortisol release are in the early morning, peaking at about 6 a.m., then falling throughout the day. This circadian variation is initiated in the hypothalamus by changing sensitivity to cortisol levels. Cortisol exerts a weaker negative feedback effect in the morning, so CRH release rises. The circadian rhythm must be taken into account when making plasma cortisol measurements.

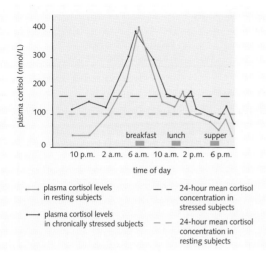

Fig. 4.8 Circadian variation in plasma cortisol in resting and chronically stressed subjects.

Actions of cortisol

Physical and psychological stressors (e.g. trauma, haemorrhage, fever) increase ACTH and cortisol secretion, which, in turn, regulate metabolic adaptations to these stimuli. This effect is very important, and cortisol deficiency can rapidly become life-threatening under stressful conditions. The response to stress is called the general adaptation syndrome (GAS), and it is divided into three phases:

Alarm reaction

A stressful stimulus causes:

- Noradrenaline release from sympathetic nerves
- Adrenaline and noradrenaline release from adrenal medulla
- Cortisol release from adrenal cortex.

Resistance

The effects of cortisol are slower to initiate, as they are dependent on transcription. However they are longer-lasting than those of adrenaline and noradrenaline; this allows the resistance to stress to be maintained. It also counteracts the effects of other hormones (e.g. insulin) to maintain substrates required to combat stress.

Exhaustion

Prolonged stress causes continued cortisol secretion, and it results in muscle wastage, immune system suppression and hyperglycaemia. Cortisol affects almost every cell in the body. The physiological effects are described in Fig. 4.9. The main actions of cortisol are:

- Increase of energy metabolite levels in the blood
- Suppression of the immune system and inhibition of allergic and inflammatory processes.

There is some overlap between the actions of mineralocorticoids and glucocorticoids. Cortisol can have mineralocorticoid actions and aldosterone can act as a glucocorticoid.

Intracellular actions of cortisol

Like all steroid hormones, cortisol acts via intracellular receptors to regulate gene expression. The receptor and genes vary between cells, and this accounts for the wide range of actions. The anti-inflammatory actions are produced by inhibiting phospholipase A_2, an enzyme that is essential for the production of prostaglandins from arachidonic acid.

Most cortisol (95%) is transported round the body bound to plasma proteins:

- 80% bound to cortisol-binding protein
- 15% bound to albumin
- 5% free and active.

Cortisol is inactivated in the liver by conjugation and then excreted from the kidney. About 1% of cortisol is excreted into the urine without metabolism. This can be detected by 24-hour urine collection to estimate blood cortisol levels.

> The immunosuppressive properties of synthetic corticosteroids ('steroids', e.g. prednisolone) are commonly employed in the treatment of autoimmune conditions and inflammatory disorders.

ANDROGENS

Androgens are sex steroids, i.e. hormones involved in the growth and function of the male and female genital tract. They also stimulate muscle growth (anabolism), hence their use as an illicit drug in sport. Androgens are made in the adrenal gland in both males and females. However, in males they account for only a small proportion of total androgen production.

Actions of adrenal androgens

Adrenal androgens are synthesized in the zona reticularis of the adrenal gland; the main adrenal androgens are:

- Dehydroepiandrosterone (DHEA)
- Androstenedione.

Androgens secreted by the adrenal glands have weak biological activity, but they are converted to more active androgens, such as testosterone, by aromatase and other enzymes in peripheral tissues.

Fig. 4.9 Physiological effects of cortisol and the symptoms of Cushing's syndrome

Process/system affected	Effect of cortisol	Related pathology in Cushing's syndrome
Carbohydrate metabolism	Raises blood glucose by stimulating gluconeogenesis and preventing glucose uptake	Hyperglycaemia and diabetes
Protein metabolism	Increases breakdown of proteins in skeletal muscle, skin and bone to release amino acids	Muscle weakness and wasting; thin easily bruising skin
Fat metabolism	Stimulates lipolysis and increases fatty acid levels in the blood	Fat redistributed to the face and trunk causing a moon face, buffalo hump, and abdominal stretch marks
Immune system	Suppresses the action and production of immune cells; inhibits the production of cytokines and antibodies	Infections, poor healing, peptic ulceration
Endocrine system	Suppresses the secretion of anterior pituitary hormones: ACTH, LH, FSH, TSH and GH	Suppression of growth in children
Nervous system	Influences fetal and neonatal neuron development; influences behaviour and cognitive function; augments the actions of the sympathetic system	Depression, insomnia, psychosis and confusion
Water metabolism	Has weak mineralocorticoid actions: raises sodium and water retention	Hypertension and heart failure
Calcium metabolism	Decreases calcium absorption from the gut; increases calcium excretion in the kidneys; increases calcium resorption from bones	Osteoporosis

ACTH, adrenocorticotrophic hormone; FSH, follicle-stimulating hormone; GH, growth hormone; LH, luteinizing hormone; TSH, thyroid-stimulating hormone.

Adrenarche

The initiation of androgen secretion from the adrenal glands is called adrenarche. It occurs a few years before puberty (about 7–9 years of age), and it is marked by maturation of the zona reticularis and a rise in plasma DHEA.

In males, the early development of the male sex organs may result from adrenal androgens released after adrenarche. In male adult life adrenal androgens account for only 5% of total activity, so they are physiologically negligible.

In the female, adrenal androgens are responsible for about 50% of total androgen activity from adrenarche to the end of life. These hormones help to promote the growth of female pubic and axillary hair.

DISORDERS OF THE ADRENAL CORTEX

The main diseases of the adrenal cortex are caused by an excess or deficiency of mineralocorticoids or glucocorticoids. There are four named diseases affecting the adrenal cortex hormones; however, they are rare diseases:

- Cushing's syndrome – chronic, excessive cortisol production
- Cushing's disease – ACTH-secreting tumour
- Conn's syndrome – aldosterone-secreting tumour
- Addison's disease – deficiency of cortisol and aldosterone.

Both Cushing's and Conn's are important endocrine causes of hypertension.

Hyperaldosteronism

Excess aldosterone production causes sodium ion and water retention with increased excretion of potassium and hydrogen ions. The main symptoms and signs (Fig. 4.10) are:

- Hypertension (high blood pressure)
- Hypokalaemia (low potassium)
- Alkalosis (raised blood pH)
- Polyuria and polydipsia (thirst)
- Muscle weakness and spasm.

Fig. 4.10 Clinical symptoms of hyperaldosteronism and hypoaldosteronism

Action of aldosterone	Hyperaldosteronism	Hypoaldosteronism
Increases plasma Na^+	Hypernatraemia rarely occurs because of other mechanisms regulating fluid volume	Loss of Na^+ is accompanied by loss of water, so plasma Na^+ concentration does not change
Decreases plasma K^+	Hypokalaemia	Hyperkalaemia
Decreases plasma H^+	Metabolic alkalosis	Mild metabolic acidosis
Maintains extracellular fluid volume	Hypertension	Volume depletion and postural hypotension

A number of blood tests are used for diagnosis:

- Urea and electrolytes (U + Es) for hypokalaemia
- Aldosterone levels (raised)
- Renin levels (variable).

Aldosterone increases blood volume, which inhibits renin secretion. If renin levels are low then the disorder is primary hyperaldosteronism, i.e. the disease originates in the adrenal glands. The adrenal glands can then be imaged by CT/MRI scanning.

Renin stimulates aldosterone release via angiotensin II, so high renin levels suggest secondary hyperaldosteronism. This disorder is external to the adrenal glands; it is a common response to heart failure and renal disease.

Primary hyperaldosteronism and Conn's syndrome

Primary hyperaldosteronism is a rare disease that is responsible for about 1% of patients with hypertension. The vast majority of primary hyperaldosteronism is caused by Conn's syndrome, in which the patients have an adenoma of the zona glomerulosa. This is discussed later in this chapter.

The triad of hypertension, hypokalaemia and alkalosis should raise the suspicion of Conn's syndrome. Conn's syndrome is the result of an adrenocortical adenoma causing primary hyperaldosteronism. Hyperaldosteronism can also be seen as part of congenital adrenal hyperplasia due to the presence of excess ACTH. Patients with Conn's syndrome have a high plasma aldosterone. They also have low plasma renin due to the effects of chronic water/salt retention. Renal artery stenosis can also cause this pattern of symptoms, but these patients have a high plasma renin.

Secondary hyperaldosteronism

Secondary hyperaldosteronism is a very common problem caused by activation of the renin–angiotensin system. The most common cause is excessive diuretic therapy, but it is also a feature of:

- Congestive heart failure
- Renal artery stenosis
- Nephritic syndrome
- Cirrhosis with ascites.

All these conditions result in decreased renal perfusion, which stimulates renin release.

Excess cortisol

Cushing's syndrome

Cushing's syndrome is a rare condition caused by a chronic excess of glucocorticoids. The disorder can be in the anterior pituitary gland or the adrenal cortex, or it may result from excess medication. It has a 5-year mortality of about 50% if it is not treated.

The symptoms and signs of Cushing's syndrome are shown in Figs 4.9 and 4.11; it is most common in adult women.

Diagnosing excess cortisol is complicated by the circadian variation in cortisol secretion. The first-line screening consists of two main tests which are employed to overcome this problem:

- Overnight dexamethasone suppression test: plasma cortisol is measured before an oral dexamethasone (a synthetic glucocorticoid) dose and then at 8 a.m. the next morning. In a normal person plasma cortisol would be suppressed.
- Twenty-four-hour urinary free cortisol: 1% of free cortisol is excreted unmetabolized, and this can be measured to give an accurate reflection of plasma cortisol.

It is important to note that 'pseudocushing's' (false positives) are seen in other diseases, e.g. depression, obesity, alcohol excess or anything that increases the rate of dexamethasone metabolism.

Fig. 4.11 Symptoms and signs of Cushing's syndrome.

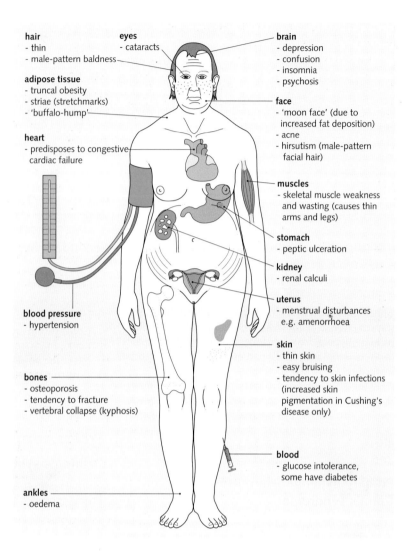

hair
- thin
- male-pattern baldness

adipose tissue
- truncal obesity
- striae (stretchmarks)
- 'buffalo-hump'

heart
- predisposes to congestive cardiac failure

blood pressure
- hypertension

bones
- osteoporosis
- tendency to fracture
- vertebral collapse (kyphosis)

ankles
- oedema

eyes
- cataracts

brain
- depression
- confusion
- insomnia
- psychosis

face
- 'moon face' (due to increased fat deposition)
- acne
- hirsutism (male-pattern facial hair)

muscles
- skeletal muscle weakness and wasting (causes thin arms and legs)

stomach
- peptic ulceration

kidney
- renal calculi

uterus
- menstrual disturbances e.g. amenorrhoea

skin
- thin skin
- easy bruising
- tendency to skin infections (increased skin pigmentation in Cushing's disease only)

blood
- glucose intolerance, some have diabetes

Second-line investigations:

- Forty-eight-hour dexamethasone suppression test: oral dexamethasone is given every 6 hours for 2 days with cortisol measured at 0 and 48 hours. In Cushing's syndrome, cortisol levels will remain elevated.
- Midnight cortisol: this is less commonly used as it requires admission and is often inaccurate. Cortisol levels are normally lowest at midnight, though it is elevated in Cushing's syndrome.

The next step is locating the source of the problem as this will determine the course of treatment.

Treatment with glucocorticoids

This is the most common cause of Cushing's syndrome. Glucocorticoids (often simply called 'steroids') are used to treat a wide range of medical conditions, usually to reduce immune reactions. These conditions include asthma, inflammatory bowel disease, rheumatoid arthritis and post-transplantation. Patients are treated with the lowest dose that will control their condition because prolonged use can cause the features of Cushing's syndrome. Inhaled steroids are used in asthma to reduce the systemic dose, especially in children, in whom growth retardation may occur.

A review of the patient's medication will locate any iatrogenic cause and, if possible, the medication needs to be gradually stopped.

Cushing's disease

Cushing's disease refers to the specific condition of excess corticosteroids as a result of pituitary adenomas. This stimulates the adrenal cortex to secrete excess cortisol, leading to bilateral enlargement of the cortex. The negative feedback that normally prevents excess ACTH release is absent in the tumour.

This type of tumour causes Cushing's syndrome with the additional sign of pigmented skin. This is due to the melanocyte-stimulating action of ACTH on the receptors for the structurally similar melanocyte-stimulating hormone (α-MSH) – formed by the same gene (POMC) that makes ACTH. Cushing's disease occurs most frequently in young adult women.

Cushing's disease is treated by surgical removal of the pituitary adenoma. This may result in panhypopituitarism (see Chapter 2 for more details).

Ectopic adrenocorticotrophic hormone production

Ectopic ACTH can be secreted by the rare, but highly malignant, small-cell anaplastic carcinoma of the lung (also called oat-cell carcinoma). This carcinoma displays the characteristics of a neuroendocrine cell despite developing from bronchial epithelium. Even more rarely, tumours of the thymus, ovary, pancreas and carcinoid tumors can secrete ACTH or CRH. The excess production is so dramatic that patients rarely exhibit features of Cushing's syndrome before death. Ectopic hormones are discussed in Chapter 10.

Neoplasia of the adrenal cortex

Benign adenoma of the adrenal cortex is relatively common, but only a small proportion secrete hormones. If cortisol is secreted, then Cushing's syndrome develops; aldosterone-secreting adenomas cause Conn's syndrome.

Adrenal adenomas are the most common cause of Cushing's syndrome in children, but they account for only 10% of adult disease. In Conn's syndrome, adenomas of the adrenal cortex are the most common cause of primary hyperaldosteronism in all age groups. Adenomas associated with either syndrome are removed surgically, but cortisol replacement is necessary due to long-term ACTH inhibition.

Carcinoma of the adrenal cortex is a very rare condition. Such carcinomas secrete vast excesses of glucocorticoids and androgens. The patient usually dies before the physical features of Cushing's syndrome develop.

The main way to localize the cause of elevated cortisol is with a plasma ACTH measurement following a 48-hour dexamethasone suppression test.

Undetectable ACTH levels indicate an adrenal tumour, which requires imaging and further investigations to locate and diagnose. If ACTH is detectable, then it is important to distinguish a Cushing's disease from ectopic ACTH production. See 'Investigations and Imaging of the Adrenal Gland'.

Deficiency of cortisol and aldosterone

Congenital adrenal hyperplasia (CAH)

ACTH controls the production of all the hormones in the zona fasciculata and the zona reticularis. Cortisol is solely responsible for negative feedback on ACTH production. Therefore, any deficiency in cortisol relieves the suppression of ACTH release and glucocorticoid, mineralocorticoid and androgen production are perturbed. The gland tends to get larger under the trophic influence of ACTH, and the condition is referred to as congenital adrenal hyperplasia (CAH).

One cause of CAH is an autosomal recessive deficiency of 21-hydroxylase. This enzyme is required for the synthesis of aldosterone and cortisol, and both hormones are deficient. Low cortisol triggers ACTH release, resulting in hyperplasia of the adrenal cortex. Low aldosterone results in salt loss and neonatal shock in some babies. The enlarged adrenal cortex secretes excess androgens, causing adrenogenital syndrome. This presents differently in each sex. It can cause ambiguous genitalia in both males and females. In males, it causes early (precocious) pseudopuberty; signs of secondary sexual development can be found by 6 months of age, but the child is not fertile. Early bone epiphyseal fusion causes short adult height.

In females, androgen excess causes masculinization (also called virilization). The symptoms are similar to those found in polycystic ovarian syndrome. They include masculine body shape, balding of temporal skull, increased muscle bulk, deepening of the voice and enlargement of the clitoris. (For greater detail, see *Crash Course Obstetrics and Gynaecology*.)

> Precocious puberty, salt-losing crisis or ambiguous genitalia all indicate a possible diagnosis of CAH. Plasma levels of 17-hydroxyprogesterone, which are raised in CAH, are used as a screen. Treatment focuses on determining the baby's gender by karotyping and replacing glucocorticoids and mineralocorticoids.

Adrenal cortex insufficiency

Adrenal cortex insufficiency tends to affect the whole adrenal cortex rather than specific layers. Accordingly, deficiencies of glucocorticoids, mineralocorticoids and androgens occur together, although clinical effects are due to cortisol and aldosterone deficiency. These effects are shown in Fig. 4.12. Hydrocortisone (cortisol) and fludrocortisone (a mineralocorticoid) therapy must be initiated before the underlying disease process is treated.

Fig. 4.12 Symptoms and signs of Addison's disease. (ACTH, adrenocorticotrophic hormone.)

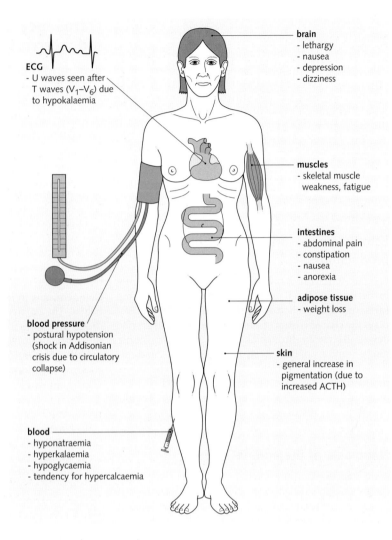

ECG
- U waves seen after T waves (V_1–V_6) due to hypokalaemia

brain
- lethargy
- nausea
- depression
- dizziness

muscles
- skeletal muscle weakness, fatigue

intestines
- abdominal pain
- constipation
- nausea
- anorexia

adipose tissue
- weight loss

skin
- general increase in pigmentation (due to increased ACTH)

blood pressure
- postural hypotension (shock in Addisonian crisis due to circulatory collapse)

blood
- hyponatraemia
- hyperkalaemia
- hypoglycaemia
- tendency for hypercalcaemia

Suspected adrenal cortex insufficiency is investigated using the ACTH stimulation test. A synthetic ACTH analogue is injected and plasma cortisol levels are measured every 30 minutes. If the cortisol levels do not rise sufficiently, then the disease is of the adrenal cortex (i.e. Addison's disease).

Addison's disease

Primary insufficiency of the adrenal cortex is called Addison's disease; it is characterized by deficient secretion of glucocorticoids and mineralocorticoids. It is a rare chronic condition caused by progressive destruction of the adrenal cortex. This destruction can result from autoimmune adrenalitis, infection (e.g. tuberculosis, fungi) or tumour. Addison's disease presents with adrenal cortex insufficiency, but the high levels of circulating ACTH can cause skin pigmentation too.

An acute exacerbation of Addison's disease is called an adrenal crisis. It is a life-threatening emergency caused by stressful events such as infection. Its presentation is the same as acute adrenocortical failure.

Acute adrenocortical failure

This is a life-threatening condition characterized by:

- Hypotensive shock
- Hypovolaemic shock
- Hypoglycaemia.

The inhibitory action of cortisol on ACTH release is important clinically. Patients treated with long-term 'steroids' cannot simply stop because ACTH release, and therefore cortisol production, would also stop. Instead, the dose must be lowered over a number of months.

The adrenal cortex can be destroyed acutely by bilateral haemorrhagic necrosis following disseminated intravascular coagulation. Essentially, blood clots block the venous drainage of the adrenal cortex, causing cell death. These clots can form following severe septicaemia. Meningococcal septicemia is the most common cause and this is called Waterhouse–Friderichsen syndrome.

A similar situation can occur if long-term high-dose steroid treatment is stopped abruptly. The prolonged treatment chronically suppresses ACTH release from the anterior pituitary gland so that no cortisol is secreted from the adrenal cortex for a number of weeks.

Secondary adrenocortical insufficiency

Disorders of the hypothalamus and anterior pituitary gland can also cause deficiency of adrenal cortex steroid hormones. Any condition that causes a reduction in CRH or ACTH release will prevent the synthesis of glucocorticoids especially. These conditions are described in more detail in Chapter 2.

HORMONES OF THE ADRENAL MEDULLA

The adrenal medulla secretes two hormones: noradrenaline and adrenaline, which are catecholamines (Fig. 4.13). Eighty per cent of catecholamine released from the adrenal glands is adrenaline. The remainder of catecholamines are released at sympathetic nerve synapses.

> Once cortisol excess has been confirmed, further tests using higher doses of dexamethasone and measuring ACTH levels can locate the source. If a 24-hour suppression test is positive and ACTH is undetectable, this suggests an adrenaloma. If the 24-hour test is positive and ACTH is high, this suggests either pituitary tumour, which can be suppressed with a 48-hour suppression test or ectopic ACTH, which cannot be suppressed with a 48-hour suppression test. CT scans are used once a source has been identified.

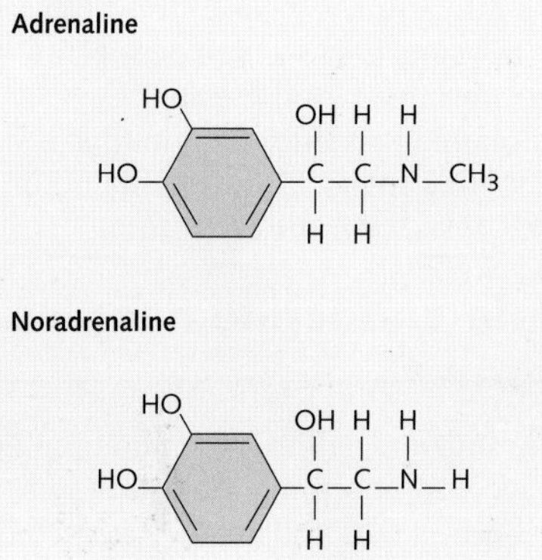

Regulation

Catecholamines are released in response to stress (e.g. exercise, pain, shock, hypoglycaemia and imminent exams). Stress stimulates an area of the hypothalamus that activates both the adrenocortical and sympatheticoadrenal systems. It receives no direct regulation from the pituitary gland. Catecholamines exert their effects over a shorter time course than cortisol.

Actions

Catecholamines from the adrenal medulla perform similar functions to direct sympathetic neuronal connections, in that they prepare the body for fight or flight. Their effects last longer than the neuronal signals, so they help to minimize the harm caused by repeated stress. Adrenaline and noradrenaline have similar effects to each other.

Their main actions are described in Fig. 4.14 (for more detail on the sympathetic nervous system, see *Crash Course Nervous System*).

Intracellular actions

Adrenal catecholamines bind to receptors in a similar manner to neuronal signals. These extracellular receptors are linked to intracellular G-proteins that initiate a signal cascade. The effect of the signal depends on the receptor present and the cell type, which are classified into alpha- and beta-adrenergic receptors.

Synthesis

Noradrenaline is synthesized from the amino acid tyrosine, which is then converted to adrenaline in response to cortisol from the adrenal cortex.

The medullary cells store catecholamines in cytoplasmic granules. They are released into blood sinusoids by exocytosis in response to acetylcholine from preganglionic sympathetic neurons.

Breakdown

Catecholamines circulate bound to albumin. They are degraded by two enzymes in the liver:

- Monoamine oxidase (MAO)
- Catechol-O-methyl transferase (COMT).

Adrenaline and noradrenaline are converted to vanillyl mandelic acid (VMA or HMMA), which is released into

Fig. 4.13 Structures of adrenaline and noradrenaline.

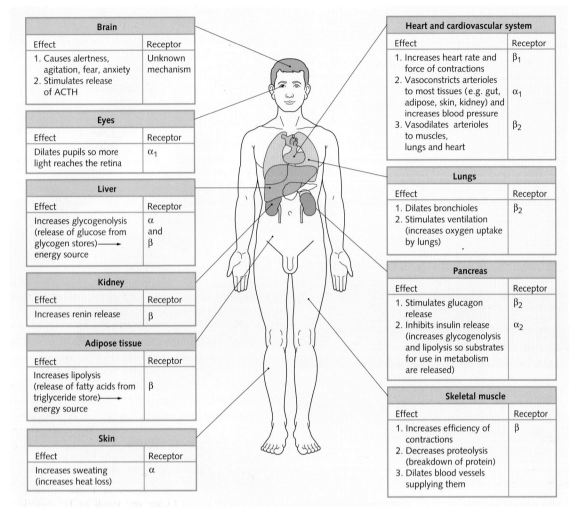

Brain	
Effect	Receptor
1. Causes alertness, agitation, fear, anxiety	Unknown mechanism
2. Stimulates release of ACTH	

Eyes	
Effect	Receptor
Dilates pupils so more light reaches the retina	α_1

Liver	
Effect	Receptor
Increases glycogenolysis (release of glucose from glycogen stores)⟶ energy source	α and β

Kidney	
Effect	Receptor
Increases renin release	β

Adipose tissue	
Effect	Receptor
Increases lipolysis (release of fatty acids from triglyceride store)⟶ energy source	β

Skin	
Effect	Receptor
Increases sweating (increases heat loss)	α

Heart and cardiovascular system	
Effect	Receptor
1. Increases heart rate and force of contractions	β_1
2. Vasoconstricts arterioles to most tissues (e.g. gut, adipose, skin, kidney) and increases blood pressure	α_1
3. Vasodilates arterioles to muscles, lungs and heart	β_2

Lungs	
Effect	Receptor
1. Dilates bronchioles	β_2
2. Stimulates ventilation (increases oxygen uptake by lungs)	

Pancreas	
Effect	Receptor
1. Stimulates glucagon release	β_2
2. Inhibits insulin release (increases glycogenolysis and lipolysis so substrates for use in metabolism are released)	α_2

Skeletal muscle	
Effect	Receptor
1. Increases efficiency of contractions	β
2. Decreases proteolysis (breakdown of protein)	
3. Dilates blood vessels supplying them	

Fig. 4.14 Physiological effects of adrenaline and noradrenaline and the receptors present in each tissue/organ. (ACTH, adrenocorticotrophic hormone.)

the urine. Urinary VMA levels are measured to detect phaeochromocytomas, a rare tumour of the adrenal medulla that is discussed below.

DISORDERS OF THE ADRENAL MEDULLA

Phaeochromocytomas

Phaeochromocytomas are very rare tumours of the catecholamine-producing cells in the adrenal medulla. They are usually benign and present in only one gland (unilateral). Adrenaline and noradrenaline are secreted in large quantities, causing severe, sporadic (paroxysmal) hypertension that can produce headaches. With time, the hypertension can become constant, leading to heart failure.

The first-choice test for diagnosing this tumour is plasma free metanephrines. Other tests include the detection of high levels of catecholamine breakdown products in the urine, e.g. VMA. It is treated by surgical excision. The surgery has a high perioperative mortality due to the unstable blood pressure.

Catecholamine-producing tumours can also develop in sympathetic ganglia. These usually occur beside the abdominal aorta, near the bifurcation.

Multiple endocrine neoplasia syndromes

A very rare autosomal dominant mutation causes inheritable phaeochromocytoma. These tumours can also develop in both glands (bilaterally) as a component of multiple endocrine neoplasia syndromes (MEN type II), described in Chapter 10.

INVESTIGATIONS AND IMAGING OF THE ADRENAL GLANDS

Investigations

Some investigations have already been discussed in this chapter. They work by detecting the levels of ACTH and cortisol. They include:

- Overnight dexamethasone suppression test – serum cortisol is measured, 1–2 mg dexamethasone is given at midnight and then a second cortisol measurement is taken at 8 a.m. Normal patients will have a decrease in both ACTH and cortisol secretion to a level of < 50 nmol/L.
- **24-hour urinary free cortisol** – urine is collected over 24 hours, with a normal value is < 280 nmol/24 h. This provides an accurate guide to plasma cortisol levels.
- **48-hour dexamethasone suppression test** – 0.5 mg/6 h PO dexamethasone is given for 2 days with cortisol measured at 0 and 48 hours. In normal patients, cortisol will fall to < 50 nmol/L and ACTH levels will drop.
- **Midnight cortisol** – this is less commonly used as it requires admission and is often inaccurate. Cortisol levels are normally lowest at midnight, though they are elevated in Cushing's syndrome.

As mentioned, these tests will help to diagnose Cushing's syndrome, but localization of the cause requires further testing.

An undetectable ACTH level indicates an adrenal tumour and requires additional testing to confirm. The main methods used are:

- **Ultrasound scanning** – the use of harmless high-frequency sound waves can determine the composition of masses. A solid mass would suggest a tumour whereas a fluid-filled mass may be a cyst.
- **Computed tomography (CT)** – produces a cross-sectional image using X-rays.

Scans of both adrenal glands are required; however, if this is unsuccessful at detecting any abnormalities then sampling from the adrenal vein to check for elevated cortisol levels may be carried out.

If ACTH levels were detectable during initial investigations then this can indicate a pituitary tumour or an ectopic ACTH-secreting tumour. To determine the difference, two tests can be used:

- **High-dose dexamethasone suppression test** – 2 mg/6 h dexamethasone is given orally for 48 hours. Measurements of cortisol in both urine and plasma are taken at 0 and 48 hours. If there is a partial or complete suppression of cortisol, this is indicative of Cushing's disease. In Cushing's disease some feedback remains so it should decrease slightly at least. An autonomous ectopic source will not be affected by the dexamethasone.
- **Corticotrophin-releasing hormone test** – 100 micrograms of human corticotrophin-releasing hormone is given intravenously. A cortisol level is measured at 2 hours. Elevated cortisol levels indicate the source of the problem is in the pituitary as CRH has no effect on an ectopic ACTH-secreting tumour.

If the tests show a pituitary source then further investigation is required to identify the exact location and direct treatment, though it is usually surgery (see Chapter 2).

If the tests indicate an ectopic ACTH-secreting tumour, then CT ± MRI of the neck, thorax and abdomen is necessary to locate any small ACTH-secreting carcinoid tumours.

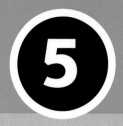

The pancreas 5

After reading this chapter you should:
- Know the relevant anatomy and developmental physiology of the pancreas and its ducts
- Understand the role of pancreatic hormones in the regulation of blood glucose
- Be able to explain the aetiology, symptoms, complications and treatment of diabetes mellitus
- Briefly discuss neoplasia of the endocrine pancreas.

The pancreas is an organ with both exocrine and endocrine functions. As an exocrine organ it is responsible for producing and secreting digestive enzymes; however, this chapter will focus on the endocrine functions of the gland. Specifically, the pancreatic control of blood glucose levels will be studied as the pancreas responds to different control mechanisms than other endocrine organs. The pancreas secretes two very important hormones that directly affect blood glucose, **insulin** and **glucagon**. However, their secretion is regulated by the levels of glucose detected by the pancreas directly and not secreted in response to hormones from the hypothalamus and pituitary gland (Fig. 5.1).

The pancreas is a flattened retroperitoneal gland located posterior and inferior to the stomach and between the stomach and duodenum. The endocrine cells of the pancreas are arranged in small clusters around the larger exocrine cell clusters, called *acini*. The endocrine clusters are called **islets of Langerhans** and within them are four types of cells, the most abundant being the β-cells which secrete insulin. Insulin is responsible for lowering blood glucose by various means including increasing cellular uptake of glucose and converting glucose to glycogen. So as food enters our gastrointestinal tract, glucose is absorbed into the body and the bloodstream. Insulin acts to prevent the glucose in the blood from rising too high and thus keeps it within tightly controlled ranges.

To prevent blood glucose from dropping too far, we have a hormone to also raise the blood glucose, **glucagon**. This is normally inhibited by insulin; however, falling blood glucose causes inhibition of insulin secretion and glucagon secretion. The glucagon acts in the reverse of many of insulin's actions, e.g. causing glucose to leave cells and enter the blood.

The most common endocrine disorder is diabetes mellitus, which is a deficiency of insulin (type 1, formerly insulin-dependent diabetes mellitus) or increased insulin resistance (type 2, formerly non-insulin-dependent diabetes mellitus). In both cases, blood glucose rises, resulting in hyperglycaemia and dehydration caused by excessive urination as water follows the movement of glucose (glycosuria) out of the body through the kidneys. Poorly controlled diabetes can lead to serious organ damage and life-threatening complications.

> Important words:
>   **Anabolism**: processes that build large molecules
>   **Catabolism**: processes that break down large molecules
>   **Glycosuria**: glucose in the urine
>   **Polyuria**: large volume of urine

ANATOMY

The pancreas is a long, flat organ that lies posterior to the stomach and extends between the duodenum and the spleen. The pancreas consists of four main parts, the head, uncinate process, body and tail (Fig. 5.2).

- The **head** lies in the C-shaped curve of the duodenum, anterior to the inferior vena cava.
- The **uncinate process** is a projection from the posterior surface of the head, forming the 'hook' of the pancreas. The superior mesenteric vessels run anterior to the uncinate process, separating it from the head.
- The **body and tail** run anteriorly over the aorta and left kidney and posterior to the stomach. The tail terminates at the hilum of the spleen. A branch of the aorta (the coeliac trunk) lies superior and gives rise to the splenic artery that lies along the upper pancreatic border.

Fig. 5.1 Hormonal regulation of blood glucose and metabolism by insulin and glucagon.

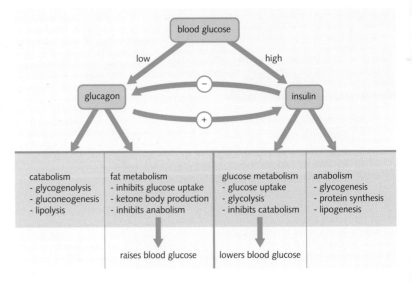

Blood, nerves and lymphatics

The body and tail of the pancreas are supplied by small branches of the splenic artery (largest branch of the coeliac trunk). The head and uncinate process are supplied by the inferior and superior, posterior and anterior pancreaticoduodenal artery, branches of the common hepatic artery. Blood drains from the pancreas through the pancreatic veins. These flow into the splenic veins and the portal vein, which leads to the liver. Lymph drains through small nodes and vessels and into the preaortic lymph nodes.

The endocrine pancreas is controlled by hormones mainly; however, some autonomic nerves do reach the pancreas. These are derived from the coeliac and superior mesenteric plexuses.

MICROSTRUCTURE

The pancreas contains two major tissue types, exocrine (enzyme-secreting) and endocrine (hormone-secreting). The endocrine cells are arranged in spherical clusters called islets of Langerhans within the exocrine tissue (Fig. 5.3). Each islet has a rich network of fenestrated capillaries; however, only 10% of endocrine cells are innervated by the autonomic nervous system.

The islets are made up of endocrine cells containing dense secretory granules. These cells are APUD (amine precursor uptake and decarboxylation) cells (see Chapter 6). There are four types of endocrine cell:

- Glucagon-secreting α-cells (20%)
- Insulin-secreting β-cells (70%)

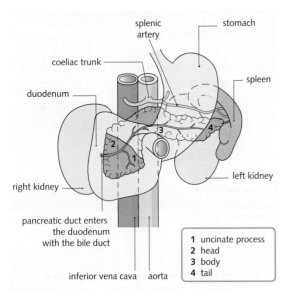

Fig. 5.2 Location of the pancreas in the retroperitoneal abdomen.

1	uncinate process
2	head
3	body
4	tail

Pancreatic duct

The digestive secretions of the pancreas are carried to the duodenum along the pancreatic duct. It begins at the tail and travels along the length of the pancreas to the head where it intersects the bile duct to become the ampulla of Vater (hepatopancreatic ampulla). This drains into the duodenum through the sphincter of Oddi, a collection of smooth muscle.

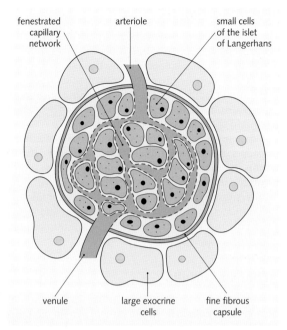

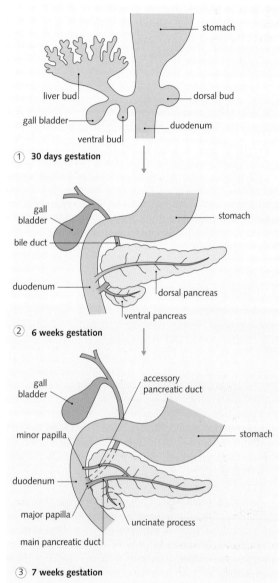

Fig. 5.3 Microstructure of the pancreas showing an islet of Langerhans surrounded by exocrine tissue.

- Somatostatin-secreting δ-cells (8%)
- Pancreatic polypeptide-secreting F-cells (2%).

Insulin and glucagon help regulate blood glucose levels. Somatostatin inhibits the release of insulin and glucagon. Pancreatic polypeptide inhibits the exocrine (i.e. non-endocrine) functions of the pancreas.

DEVELOPMENT

The pancreas is an endodermal structure that develops from two buds derived from the foregut:

- Dorsal bud – the larger bud that forms the majority of the gland
- Ventral bud – the smaller bud from the right side near the bile duct.

The ventral bud rotates behind the duodenum, along with the bile duct, to lie posterior to the dorsal bud. This smaller ventral bud forms the uncinate process as it fuses with the larger dorsal bud. The ducts usually fuse so that the end of the pancreatic duct is formed from the smaller ventral bud. The duct of the dorsal bud may persist as the accessory pancreatic duct. This sequence is shown in Fig. 5.4.

All the pancreatic cells are thought to arise from a single endodermal precursor. *Notch*, *TGF-beta* and *sonic hedgehog* are key genes in determining whether endodermal calls become pancreatic precursors, whether these cells differentiate into exocrine or endocrine cells and, finally, which islet cell lineage is followed. Other

Fig. 5.4 Embryological development of the pancreas.

factors, including cell adhesion molecules (integrins and NCAMs) and proteolytic enzymes (i.e. matrix metalloproteinases), determine how the precursor cells migrate through the developing pancreas.

HORMONES

Insulin

Insulin is a hormone that promotes the uptake, storage and use of glucose. The beta islet cells secrete insulin when they detect high blood glucose levels. As glucose levels fall a few hours after a meal, insulin secretion is reduced. The stored glucose can then be released to maintain blood levels. Insulin secretion never ceases completely; there is always a basal level of insulin in the blood.

Synthesis

Insulin is a polypeptide hormone consisting of two short chains (A and B) linked by disulphide bonds. A single gene controls the production of preproinsulin, which is broken down to form proinsulin. Further cleavage occurs within the secretory vesicles, resulting in two molecules: insulin and C-peptide. Since equimolar insulin and C-peptide are produced, C-peptide acts as a useful marker for β-cell activity in diabetics who receive insulin treatment.

Control of insulin secretion

Insulin secretion is controlled directly by detecting blood glucose levels. Glucose and other metabolites (e.g. amino acids and triglycerides, etc.) diffuse into the beta islet cells, leading to increased ATP production. The raised intracellular ATP levels inhibit membrane-bound potassium channels, causing beta cell depolarization. This causes voltage-sensitive calcium channels to open, raising intracellular calcium. This rise promotes secretion of insulin in a biphasic pattern: the immediate release of preformed insulin, lasting less than a minute, and then a sustained release of newly formed insulin (Fig. 5.5). Normal daily adult production of insulin is 45–50 units.

Although metabolite concentrations are the main regulators of insulin release, a number of other stimulants can also affect this pathway (Fig. 5.6). These stimuli can have either an inhibitory or stimulating effect on plasma insulin levels but never reduce them completely.

Insulin receptors

The insulin receptor consists of an alpha subunit, which is extracellular, and an intracytoplasmic beta subunit, which has tyrosine kinase activity. It must act via cell-surface receptors because it is a polypeptide hormone and cannot readily cross the cell membrane. Insulin receptors are present in most cells, and they can be sequestered into the cell to inactivate them.

When insulin binds to the tyrosine kinase receptors, it causes phosphorylation of tyrosine side chains within the receptor. The phosphorylated receptor forms a complex with and phosphorylates insulin receptor substrate 1 (IRS-1). This activated molecule then initiates a cascade of phosphorylation and aggregation of other proteins to bring about the intracellular effects of insulin.

Actions of insulin

Insulin has an anabolic effect; it promotes the synthesis of larger molecules. The stimulation of insulin receptors regulates a variety of enzymes concerned with metabolites. The specific enzymes vary between cells (Fig. 5.7), but the overall effects are:

- Increased uptake of metabolites
- Conversion of metabolites to stored forms (this is an anabolic effect)
- Decreased breakdown of stored metabolites
- Recruitment of glucose channels to the cell membranes (e.g. GLUT 4)
- Use of glucose for energy over other metabolites.

Breakdown of insulin

Circulatory insulin has a half-life of approximately 5 minutes; however, proinsulin (released with insulin) has a longer half-life, approximately 20 minutes. Insulin is broken down primarily in the kidney and liver as well as the placenta but almost every tissue can break it down.

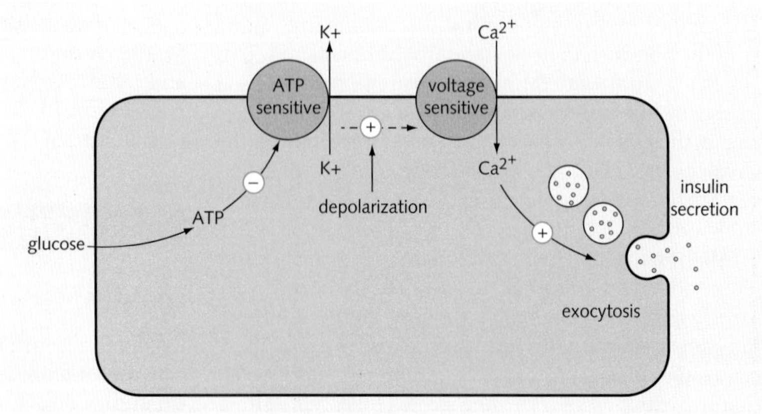

Fig. 5.5 Intracellular stimulation of insulin secretion by glucose.

Fig. 5.6 Factors controlling insulin and glucagon secretion

	Insulin		Glucagon	
	Stimulants	**Inhibitors**	**Stimulants**	**Inhibitors**
Blood glucose	High	Low	Low	High
Metabolites	Amino acids, fatty acids and ketones	–	Amino acids	Fatty acids and ketones
Hormones	Glucagon, some gastrointestinal tract peptides, growth hormone, adrenocorticotrophic hormone (ACTH), thyroid-stimulating hormone (TSH)	Adrenaline, somatostatin	Adrenaline, some gastrointestinal tract peptides	Insulin, somato-statin
Innervation	Parasympathetic	Sympathetic	Parasympathetic and sympathetic	–
Other	–	Hypocalcaemia	–	–

Fig. 5.7 Metabolic effects of insulin on target cells

Target cells	Action of insulin
Muscle cells and many other cells	Stimulates glucose uptake
	Stimulates glycogenesis (glucose→glycogen)
	Stimulates glycolysis (glucose→energy)
	Stimulates amino acid uptake and protein synthesis
	Inhibits glycogenolysis (glycogen→glucose)
	Inhibits proteolysis (protein→amino acids)
Adipose cells	Stimulates glucose uptake
	Stimulates lipogenesis (glucose→fatty acids)
	Inhibits lipolysis (fatty acids→energy)
Liver cells	Stimulates glycogenesis (glucose→glycogen)
	Inhibits glycogenolysis (glycogen→glucose)
	Inhibits gluconeogenesis (amino acids→glucose)
Hypothalamus	May stimulate satiety (fullness)

Glucagon

Glucagon is synthesized in the pancreatic α cells and is secreted in response to low levels of metabolites, resulting in a release of stored metabolites. In many respects, glucagon has the opposite effect to insulin and functions to ensure there is an adequate supply of energy between meals. The most important cause for glucagon secretion is falling glucose; however, a number of other factors stimulate its release (Fig. 5.6).

Synthesis and actions

Glucagon is a single-chain polypeptide hormone formed from a larger precursor in a manner similar to insulin. The precursor is pre-proglucagon, which is cleaved in the storage vesicles to yield proglucagon and, finally, glucagon and the glucagon-like peptides.

Glucagon is a catabolic hormone; it promotes the breakdown of large molecules. Glucagon binds to G-protein-coupled receptor on the cell membrane, and cAMP acts as a second messenger to initiate a cascade effect. Its effects vary between tissues (Fig. 5.8) but broadly its actions are:

- Inhibition of glucose and amino acid uptake
- Breakdown of stored metabolites into useable metabolites (catabolism)
- Use of fatty acids for energy over other metabolites
- Promotes hepatic output of ketone bodies.

ENDOCRINE CONTROL OF GLUCOSE HOMEOSTASIS

All cells in the body are capable of using glucose as an energy source by the process of glycolysis. Most cells can also use fatty acids with two important exceptions:

- Neurons (particularly the CNS), although they can adapt to use ketone bodies
- Blood cells.

If blood glucose levels drop too low (hypoglycaemia) then the brain is starved of energy. If levels rise too high (hyperglycaemia) then glucose can become toxic. Blood glucose is tightly controlled within narrow limits to prevent either scenario. Fasting glucose levels are normally 3.5–5.5 mmol/L.

For glucose levels to be maintained (glucose homeostasis), the body must be able to increase or decrease these levels in response to changes. There are a number of ways that the body can respond (Fig. 5.9). The liver is especially important in raising blood glucose.

Insulin and glucagon

Glucose homeostasis is maintained by the interplay between insulin and glucagon. These two hormones act as antagonists of each other because they are secreted under opposing conditions (Fig. 5.10).

- Insulin lowers blood glucose by stimulating uptake, metabolism and anabolism. It also inhibits the actions of glucagon.
- Glucagon raises blood glucose by stimulating gluconeogenesis (synthesis of glucose from amino acids) and glycogenolysis (breakdown of glycogen to release glucose). It also inhibits the actions of insulin but stimulates insulin secretion.

Insulin is the only hormone that lowers blood glucose levels but a number of hormones, including glucagon and adrenaline (epinephrine), can raise them.

Fig. 5.8 Metabolic effects of glucagon on target cells	
Target cells	**Action of glucagon**
Muscle cells and many other cells	Stimulates glycogenolysis (glycogen→glucose)
	Inhibits glucose uptake
	Inhibits glycolysis (glucose→energy)
	Inhibits amino acid uptake and protein synthesis
Adipose cells	Stimulates lipolysis (fatty acids→energy)
Liver cells	Stimulates glycogenolysis (glycogen→glucose)
	Stimulates gluconeogenesis (amino acids→glucose)
	Stimulates ketogenesis (fatty acids→ketone bodies)

Fig. 5.9 Responses that alter blood glucose levels

Responses that raise blood glucose	Responses that lower blood glucose
Ingestion of glucose in the diet	Increased uptake in cells
Gluconeogenesis – the irreversible conversion of amino acids to glucose (liver)	Metabolism to produce energy
Glycogenolysis – the reversible breakdown of glycogen to release glucose (liver)	Glycogenesis – the reversible conversion of glucose to glycogen
	Lipogenesis – the irreversible conversion of glucose to fatty acids

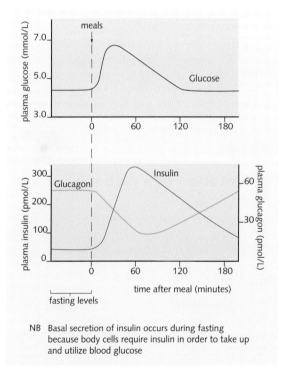

NB Basal secretion of insulin occurs during fasting because body cells require insulin in order to take up and utilize blood glucose

Fig. 5.10 Changes in blood levels of glucose, insulin and glucagon after a carbohydrate-rich meal.

Other hormones

Three non-pancreatic hormones also significantly increase blood glucose:

- Adrenaline – released in response to stress; it inhibits insulin.
- Cortisol – released in response to stress; it reduces sensitivity to insulin, which explains the diabetes seen in Cushing's patients.

- Growth hormone – released at night; it reduces sensitivity to insulin.

All three hormones can stimulate glycogenolysis and gluconeogenesis to raise blood glucose levels directly. Neural signals and other hormones can cause less significant rises in blood glucose.

Hyperglycaemia

Hyperglycaemia is an excess of glucose in the blood; it is defined as a fasting concentrations >7.8 mmol/L. This can occur in:

- Diabetes mellitus – a common disease caused by insulin deficiency or insulin resistance (reduced sensitivity)
- Glucagonoma – a very rare tumour of the α cells that secrete glucagon.

Hypoglycaemia

Hypoglycaemia is a deficiency of blood glucose defined as a concentration <2.5 mmol/L. It can result from a variety of reasons, including:

- Taking oral hypoglycaemics (e.g. sulphonylurea) or too much insulin
- Alcohol (binge or heavy drinking). This is very important to remember when assessing someone who you think is drunk, as hypoglycaemia can mimic drunkenness as well as be caused by it
- Certain medications, e.g. quinine, salicylates or propanolol
- Inappropriate levels of exercise or food intake. Type 1 diabetics control their blood glucose by balancing insulin dosage, food intake and energy expended through exercise
- Rare cases include liver, kidney, pancreas or thyroid disease. Another cause is advanced insulin-secreting tumours elsewhere in the body.

DIABETES MELLITUS

Types of diabetes mellitus

Diabetes mellitus (DM) may be primary or secondary; however, only 1–2% of presenting cases are as a result of secondary causes (Fig. 5.11). Secondary causes are important to catch as they are often treatable.

DM is caused by insulin deficiency or insulin resistance (reduced sensitivity) and results in chronic hyperglycaemia and metabolic abnormalities. This is a very important disorder to understand as it is on the rise, currently affecting 5.4% of the population of England. The main types of DM are:

- Type 1 – caused by insulin deficiency
- Type 2 – caused by insulin insufficiency and/or resistance
- Gestational diabetes resulting from pregnancy.

Type 1 DM

Type 1 DM is caused by autoimmune destruction of the β-islet cells resulting in insulin deficiency. Tests reveal autoantibodies in the blood of these patients in the early years of life, long before clinical presentation. Type 1 DM has a peak incidence during puberty but a variant form of type 1 DM called latent autoimmune diabetes of adults (LADA) can occur at any age.

Type 1 DM has a genetic association with changes in the human leucocyte antigen (HLA) genes. In a pair of identical twins, when one develops type 1 DM the other has a 30–50% chance of developing it also. This points to the development of the condition being multifactorial.

Type 2 DM

Type 2 DM used to be viewed as a disease of the elderly but it is gradually rising in younger patients, mainly those who are obese. It results from a decreased sensitivity to insulin, or insulin insufficiency (compared to deficiency in type 1 DM) or a combination of the two. In type 2 DM, the body develops a resistance to insulin over time and as such the body tries to compensate by increasing insulin secretion. This continues over a period of several years until eventually the β-islet cells fail and insulin secretion completely stops. Patients with type 2 DM may present before or after the point when insulin secretion ceases and this will affect their treatment.

Family history is very important, with approximately 50% concordance in identical twins.

Maturity-onset diabetes of the young (MODY)

This is a different form of diabetes to the others and refers to several hereditary forms of diabetes caused by mutations in an autosomal dominant gene, which disrupts insulin production. MODY is caused by at least nine different gene defects and labelled MODY 1, MODY 2, etc. MODY 2 and MODY 3 are the most common forms. Around 2% of all diabetes cases are caused by MODY gene defects. MODY is sometimes compared to type 2 diabetes, and shares some type 2 diabetes symptoms. However, MODY is not linked to obesity, and typical MODY patients are young and not necessarily overweight. The severity of the different types varies considerably.

Presentation of a diabetic patient

As discussed, insulin has an important role in glucose homeostasis and metabolic regulation. As such DM can present in a variety of ways, though there are some differences in how each type can present.

Type 1 DM

Typically patients with undiagnosed type 1 DM present with rapid onset of complaints (approximately 2–6-week history, sometimes days). However it is important

Fig. 5.11 Secondary causes of diabetes
Endocrine – Cushing's syndrome, thyrotoxicosis, phaechromocytoma, acromegaly, glucagonoma
Liver – Cirrhosis
Pancreas – Chronic pancreatitis, pancreatectomy, haemochromatosis, pancreatic carcinoma, cystic fibrosis
Drug-induced – Thiazide diuretics, corticosteroid use
Receptor anomalies – Acanthosis nigricans, congenital lipodystrophy
Genetic syndromes – Friedreich's ataxia, dystrophia myotonica

to realize that both types of DM can present with the following symptoms/signs:

- Polyuria – blood glucose exceeds the threshold for renal reabsorption resulting in osmotic diuresis
- Dehydration/thirst – as a result of excess fluid and electrolyte loss
- Weight loss – loss of fluid and accelerated fat and muscle breakdown secondary to insulin deficiency.

Additionally a patient, particularly a young patient, can present with the early signs of diabetic ketoacidosis. Signs of starvation are also important to note as they appear mainly in type 1 DM; both signs are discussed later.

Type 2 DM

As mentioned, the main difference in presentation between a patient with type 1 and one with type 2 DM is the history of the complaint. Type 1 DM typically presents as an acute problem, whereas type 2 usually has a much more gradual onset, with chronic problems developing over several months or years. The presenting complaint is typically related to a complication brought on by years of worsening hyperglycaemia. The signs/symptoms typically seen are:

- Lethargy/tiredness
- Blurred vision
- Tingling and numbness in the feet
- Impotence
- Boils
- Pruritus vulvae.

Other key presenting symptoms to be aware of are discussed below.

Symptoms of hyperglycaemia

Hyperglycaemia causes dehydration because glucose is an osmotically active substance, i.e. it draws water towards it. In hyperglycaemia, glucose concentration is high in the blood and low in the cells so the cells become dehydrated. The excess glucose is also excreted by the kidney and again water follows this movement. Excess water is lost from the body along with the electrolytes. The symptoms are summarized in Fig. 5.12.

Symptoms of hypoglycaemia

In hypoglycaemia the body has insufficient glucose to carry out its normal functions. The brain relies heavily on blood glucose as it has no glucose stores of its own; therefore, even mild hypoglycaemia can cause symptoms. The early signs/symptoms of mild hypoglycaemia include:

- Feeling hungry
- Trembling or shakiness
- Sweating
- Anxiety or irritability
- Going pale
- Tachycardia or palpitations
- Tingling in the extremities or lips.

Fig. 5.12 Symptoms of diabetes

Symptoms due to hyperglycaemia	Symptoms due to starvation	Symptoms due to ketoacidosis	Symptoms due to chronic complications
Polyuria (increased urine volume)	Weight loss	Vomiting	Decreased visual acuity
Glycosuria (glucose in the urine)	Wasting	Acetone smell on the breath	Reduced sensation in the limbs
Polydipsia (thirst)	Weakness	Ketonuria, polyuria and dehydration	Proteinuria
Tiredness		Hyperventilation	Oedema
Tendency to infections		Reduced consciousness	Intermittent claudication
Dehydration (loose skin, hypotension and tachycardia)		Convulsions	Ischaemic heart disease
Coma		Coma	Hypertension

Someone suffering from severe hypoglycaemia can resemble someone who is drunk, so this should be kept in mind when assessing patients with these symptoms. They can have difficulty concentrating, be confused and behave in a disorderly or irrational manner.

Symptoms of starvation

A lack of insulin over a protracted period of time can cause the body to enter into a state of starvation. The excess circulating glucose, caused by raised glucagon, cannot enter the cells due to the lack of insulin. This causes muscle and adipose tissue to be broken down to release metabolites. The symptoms are listed in Fig. 5.12.

Preparations of insulin vary in their duration of action and regimens are adapted according to the patient's lifestyle and requirements. Typically, long-acting insulin (Lente) is given in the morning and at night to provide basal insulin requirements and short-acting insulin is administered 15 minutes prior to a meal to cope with the postprandial hyperglycaemia. If control is poor in the morning on this regimen then night-time insulin (Lente) is adjusted. Insulin Lispro is a very rapidly acting insulin preparation that can be used before a meal.

Diabetic ketoacidosis (DKA)

This can be a dangerous and life-threatening complication of type 1 diabetes. If a patient with type 2 diabetes develops DKA, their diagnosis may need to be changed from type 2 diabetes to type 1 diabetes except in certain circumstances described below. It can present with subtle symptoms but can rapidly progress if not treated correctly.

Mechanism of DKA

In the absence of insulin, the body is unable to use glucose for energy and fatty acids are released from adipose tissue. These are converted to ketone bodies (acetoacetate and β-hydroxybutyrate) by the liver. The ketone bodies are acidic and result in a metabolic acidosis.

The excess glucose (and the ketones) causes osmotic diuresis as water and solutes are pulled into the urine, which makes the patient dehydrated.

In type 1 diabetes there is a complete absence of insulin but in type 2, insulin secretion may still be occurring, which can suppress ketogenesis. However, extreme insulin resistance can lead to the formation of ketones as there is evidence to suggest that high levels of glucose actually suppress insulin secretion, a phenomenon called glucotoxicity. The mechanism for this is yet to be fully determined. This means that patients with type 2 DM may present in a state known as Hyperosmolar Hyperglycaemic State, or HHS (previously known as HyperOsmolar

Non-Ketotic or HONK). Like DKA it is a life-threatening condition and can present with similar symptoms.

Symptoms of DKA

Patients usually present with a history of the classic symptoms of diabetes along with a few additional signs/symptoms:

- Polyuria
- Excessive thirst
- Lethargy
- Anorexia
- Hyperventilation
- Ketotic breath (sweet smelling of pear drops)
- Dehydration
- Vomiting
- Abdominal pain
- Coma.

Complications of diabetes

Both types of diabetes can produce complications despite treatment; however, good glucose control lowers the risk of developing severe complications. Chronic complications are grouped according to the size of blood vessel they affect:

- Macrovascular – large vessel disease due to accelerated atherosclerosis
- Microvascular – small vessel disease due to hyaline arteriosclerosis.

Macrovascular complications

Diabetes is a major risk factor for the development of atherosclerosis. This results from raised fatty-acid levels (hyperlipidaemia) caused by low insulin levels. Atheroma develops more rapidly and more severely than in non-diabetics, and it can block arteries, causing ischaemia and a high risk of infarction. The major sites of macrovascular disease (Fig. 5.13) are:

- The brain – the risk of stroke is twice as likely
- The heart – the risk of myocardial infarction is 3–5 times greater
- The kidneys – renal artery stenosis and hypertension
- The legs – gangrene, leading to amputation is 50 times more likely.

Microvascular complications

While atherosclerosis develops in major arteries, the smaller arterioles and capillaries are at risk of hyaline arteriolosclerosis. This is characterized by thickening of the vessel wall and basement membrane. The vessel lumen is reduced, causing localized ischaemia. Furthermore, the vessel loses integrity, allowing blood and exudates to leak out. There are four main patterns of

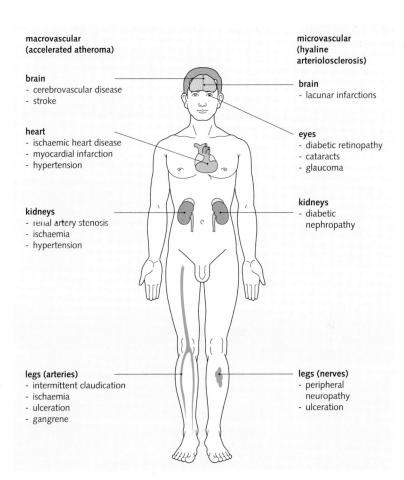

macrovascular
(accelerated atheroma)

brain
- cerebrovascular disease
- stroke

heart
- ischaemic heart disease
- myocardial infarction
- hypertension

kidneys
- renal artery stenosis
- ischaemia
- hypertension

legs (arteries)
- intermittent claudication
- ischaemia
- ulceration
- gangrene

microvascular
(hyaline
arteriolosclerosis)

brain
- lacunar infarctions

eyes
- diabetic retinopathy
- cataracts
- glaucoma

kidneys
- diabetic
  nephropathy

legs (nerves)
- peripheral
  neuropathy
- ulceration

Fig. 5.13 Chronic complications of diabetes mellitus.

microvascular disease (Fig. 5.13). Diabetic retinopathy remains one of the most common causes of blindness in people aged 30–65 years old.

Diagnosis

Normal blood glucose levels are normally 3.5–5.5 mmol/L after an overnight fast. The most up-to-date NICE guidelines for diabetes are given below.

One of the tests carried out in the diagnosis is a 2-hour fasting glucose level measurement. The patient's plasma glucose is measured, then the patient ingests a 75-g glucose preparation and 2 hours later, plasma glucose is measured again. The diagnostic criteria for diabetes are:

- A fasting plasma glucose level of ≥ 7.0 mmol/L (126 mg/dL) **OR**
- A 2-hour plasma glucose level of ≥ 11.1 mmol/L (200 mg/dL).

The report also provides diagnostic criteria for impaired glucose tolerance (IGT) and impaired fasting glucose (IFG), which if diagnosed can provide a warning to possible future development of diabetes. The criteria for IGT are:

- A 2-hour plasma glucose level of ≥ 7.8 mmol/L and < 11.1 mmol/L (140 mg/dL and 200 mg/dL).

The criteria for IFG are:

- A fasting plasma glucose level between 6.1 and 6.9 mmol/L (110 mg/dL and 125 mg/dL).

Another important and easy test is a urine dipstick for glucose. Glycosuria (glucose in the urine) can indicate diabetes and requires further investigations. Currently there are no guidelines on the use of the blood test HbA1c as a diagnostic tool for diabetes. However, HbA1c is now being considered as a diagnostic tool globally.

Additional test for autoantibodies and measuring for C-peptide deficiency can help determine decline in β-islet cell function, which is useful in discriminating type 1 from type 2 diabetes. However, there are no guidelines on its use as a diagnostic tool for diabetes.

The information on diagnosis has been adapted, with permission, from the National Institute for Health and Clinical Excellence (2004) 'CG 15 Type 1 diabetes: diagnosis and management of type 1 diabetes in children, young people and adults'. London: NICE. Available from www.nice.org.uk.

MANAGEMENT OF DIABETES

The key to successful management of diabetes relies largely on educating both the patient and, where appropriate, the patient's family on the treatment involved. It is essential to make sure they understand that the condition requires lifelong control. The management varies between individuals to a degree and between the different forms of diabetes. There is, however, some overlap.

Diet

Dietary advice should be given to help regulate blood glucose and minimize the risk of developing complications. Dietary intake should be distributed as follows:

- Carbohydrates – more than 50%
- Protein – 10–15%
- Fat – 30–35%.

    Additional advice to give patients includes:

- Avoid rapidly absorbing carbohydrates (e.g. glucose) to prevent hyperglycaemia.
- Eat regular, small meals to prevent hypoglycaemia.
- Control calorie intake to lose/stabilize weight (especially type 2).
- Eat a low-fat, healthy diet to reduce atherosclerosis.
- Avoid smoking, recreational drugs and alcohol (eating carbohydrates before and after drinking reduces risk of hypoglycaemic attack).
- Regular exercise can improve insulin sensitivity but adjustments to insulin dosage and food intake are vital.

Monitoring glucose control

Diabetics monitor their blood glucose levels regularly to help with both short- and long-term control. The following tests are available:

- Urine testing – not recommended for glucose monitoring as it is ineffective and associated with a low patient satisfaction. Useful for monitoring for ketonuria.
- Capillary blood spot testing – most commonly used monitoring device for diabetics. Modern devices are very simple to use and it gives an instant blood glucose level.
- Glycosylated haemoglobin (HbA1c) – glucose binds directly and irreversibly to haemoglobin to form HbA1c. The proportion of HbA1c in the blood gives a measure of glucose control over the previous 3 months (i.e. the approximate lifespan of a red blood cell). It is commonly performed on diabetics to help long-term management plans.

Management of type 1 DM

The main method of management is with subcutaneous insulin injections, regular glucose monitoring and a good diet.

Subcutaneous insulin injections

Insulin must be injected because it is inactivated if taken orally. Typically the injection is given in the thigh or lower abdomen. It is important to rotate through the sites with each injection as only using one site will lead to lipohypertrophy (build up of fatty tissue at the site of injection) or, less commonly, lipoatrophy (loss of adipose tissue at the site). This can be unsightly and can lead to erratic insulin absorption and poor blood glucose control.

The insulin forms currently being marketed are harvested from genetically altered bacteria, which produce recombinant human insulin. This method greatly reduces any adverse immune responses and complications in patients.

There are a variety of insulin regimens, each tailored to suit the individual, to allow the best blood glucose management. However, there are three basic regimens:

- One injection a day usually a long- or intermediate-acting insulin
- Two insulin injections per day – with a mix of rapid- or short-acting insulin with intermediate-acting insulin
- Multiple daily injection regimen – injections of rapid- or short-acting insulin are taken before meals, together with one or more separate daily injections of intermediate-acting or long-acting insulin
- Continuous subcutaneous insulin infusion (insulin pump therapy) – a programmable pump and insulin storage reservoir that gives regular or continuous insulin infusions.

Current guidelines recommend different management plans depending on age.

- Preschool and primary school children should be place on individualized treatment regimens to maximize glycaemic control.
- Young people should be offered multiple daily injection regimens to maximize glycaemic control. This should be offered only as part of a package of care that includes continuing education, dietary management, instruction on the use of insulin and blood glucose monitoring, etc.
- Adults with type 1 diabetes should have access to the types of insulin that they find allows them optimal well-being.

Management of type 2 DM

Type 2 diabetes can be managed with lifestyle changes alone for some time depending on the severity of the disease at the time of presentation. However, as type

2 DM is a chronic, progressive disorder, pharmacological treatment will become part of a patient's management at some point. Recent studies advocate intensive therapy to aggressively manage blood glucose in type 2 diabetes.

Oral hypoglycaemic agents

These are the front-line treatment in those patients who still have functioning insulin secretion. A number of medications are available:

- Biguanides – increase peripheral glucose uptake and reduce glucose output from the liver. Their mechanism of action is not fully understood. Side effects include nausea, diarrhoea and lactic acidosis. They are the first line of most treatments; the only available biguanide is metformin.
- Sulphonylureas – stimulate β-cells by inhibiting the membrane-bound K^+ channel; the resulting depolarization causes insulin release side effects including weight gain and hypoglycaemia. This is usually the second line of treatment. Examples of this class of drugs are gliclazide and glimepiride.
- Acarbose inhibits intestinal enzymes, preventing the digestion of starch, resulting in a slower rise in blood glucose after a meal. Side effects include flatulence and diarrhoea.
- Thiazolidinediones – drugs that promote insulin sensitivity, and they are usually used in combination with other drugs. They are contraindicated in people with heart failure (they cause fluid retention) or at higher risk of fractures. They are recommended as a substitute second-line treatment instead of either metformin or sulphonylureas. The only available glitazone is pioglitazone
- Gliptins, also called dipeptidyl peptidase 4 inhibitors (DPP-4) – relatively new drug. Their mechanism of action is not fully understood and is thought to be as a result of increased incretin (GLP-1 and GIP) levels, which results in inhibited glucagon, increased insulin secretion and therefore lower blood glucose. Side effects include headaches, nausea and nasopharyngitis. Its use as an additional treatment after metformin or sulphonylureas is recommended. Currently sitagliptin and vildagliptin are available for use.

- GLP-1/Incretin mimetic – *administered via injection*. It acts to promote insulin secretion, reduces glucagon activity and slows glucose absorption in the gut. Given as a third-level therapy in people with a $BMI \geq 35.0$ kg/m^2 or where insulin administration would have occupational implications. Side effects include nausea, vomiting, diarrhoea and stomach pain.

Patients with type 2 diabetes are often treated with insulin in a similar manner to those with type 1. This does not mean that they have developed type 1. Insulin treatment helps to control blood glucose, which has been proven to reduce complications.

EXAMINATION OF THE DIABETIC PATIENT

The presentation of the patient determines the examinations that will be preformed. All newly diagnosed diabetics will undergo a series of general examinations (Fig. 5.14) and investigations that will be checked on a regular basis as part of good clinical practice and ongoing management.

Undiagnosed patients with type 1 diabetes will have a fairly typical presentation and will undergo a series of routine tests to determine the cause of their symptoms. They are not likely to require an examination in the clinical setting unless they present with an associated problem. Possible presenting complaints that would require additional examination:

- Thrush – GU examination
- Altered sensation – sensory examination
- Abdominal pain – abdominal examination
- Palpitations – cardiovascular examination.

Undiagnosed type 2 diabetics will present with a specific problem and associated symptoms that will point to the diagnosis. Possible presenting complaints and the associated examinations:

Fig. 5.14 Examination of a newly diagnosed diabetic	
General	Height, weight, BMI
Cardiovascular	Blood pressure, heart rate, peripheral pulses
Neurological	Peripheral sensation
Skin	Sign of skin infections, signs of hyperlipidaemia, check for ulcers

- Visual problems – ophthalmoscopy, visual fields and acuity
- 'Pins and needles/altered sensation – CNS examination noting extent of change
- Ulcers – foot examination and peripheral pulses
- Thrush – GU examination.

Hypoglycaemia in non-diabetic patients

Most people should be able to tolerate fasting for several days without developing hypoglycaemia. If a patient is unable to do so then the mnemonic 'EXPLAIN' can be useful:

- **EX**ogenous drugs (e.g. alcohol and insulin)
- **P**ituitary insufficiency, growth hormone deficiency
- **L**iver failure or defective liver enzymes
- **A**ddison's disease – deficiency of cortisol that raises blood glucose levels (Autoimmune causes)
- **I**nsulinomas – a type of islet cell tumour (see below)
- **N**on-pancreatic tumour – by ectopic insulin secretion or excess glucose consumption.

Diabetes, pancreatic transplants and stem cells

Type 1 diabetes results from autoimmune destruction of beta islet cells and type 2 can be as a result of those cells failing to produce enough insulin to match rising resistance, possibly leading to them dying out.

Understanding the molecular biology of pancreatic development and the pathology of diabetes is the main way of advancing the management and possibly even treatment of diabetes. Transplantation of islet cells is

an established protocol but the current supply of tissue is outstripped by demand. Our understanding of certain factors (e.g. *Notch, sonic hedgehog* and *TGF-beta*) is aimed at devising a means to create new beta islet cells or regenerate existing cells in vivo. This could overcome the tissue shortage as well as immunological complications of transplantation. Alternatively, the use of stem cells to re-grow specific cells or entire organs is developing and this could be another treatment in the future (Fig. 5.15).

OTHER DISORDERS OF THE PANCREAS

Endocrine pancreatic neoplasia

Tumours of the endocrine cells in the pancreas are called islet cell tumours; they are usually benign and solitary, but they often secrete a specific hormone. Tumours are named according to the hormone they secrete:

- Insulinomas are the most common type of islet cell tumour. The excess insulin that they secrete causes severe hypoglycaemic attacks, which can lead to coma.
- Glucagonomas are very rare tumours that secrete glucagon. They are often asymptomatic, but they may cause diabetes mellitus.

Extremely infrequently, islet cell tumours can secrete other hormones, such as gastrin in Zollinger–Ellison syndrome. Other rare tumours can produce vasoactive intestinal polypeptide (VIP) or adrenocorticotrophic hormone (ACTH).

Fig. 5.15 The action of leptin on fertility. (FSH, follicle-stimulating hormone; GnRH, gonadotrophin-releasing hormone; LH, luteinizing hormone.)

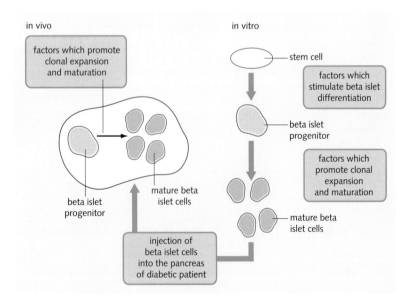

Metabolic syndrome/Syndrome X

Type 2 diabetes is often associated with hyperglycaemia, hyperinsulinaemia, dyslipidaemia, hypertension and central obesity (adipose tissue in an abdominal distribution). This collection of problems is collectively referred to as the metabolic syndrome and is associated with an increased risk of stroke and coronary heart disease, which may be the result of hypertriglyceridaemia or hyperinsulinaemia. There are several theories about why these factors cluster. Suggestions include simple genetic linkage, whilst others think that insulin resistance is the initiating event, as it drives the synthesis of triglycerides and very-low-density lipoproteins (VLDL), which in turn lead to obesity and coronary vascular disease. Alternatively, as adipose tissue produces several hormones that mediate insulin sensitivity, it may be obesity itself which creates the metabolic syndrome. Growing adipocytes produce tumour necrosis factor (TNF-α), which increases insulin resistance. Adiponectin is produced by adipose tissue and decreases insulin resistance but its levels decrease with obesity. Whilst the identification of a single underlying cause remains elusive, the metabolic syndrome serves to highlight the importance of treating other cardiac risk factors in diabetes patients.

Up and coming hormones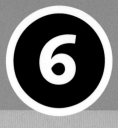

6

Objectives

By the end of this chapter you should be able to:
- Recall the constituents of the gut–brain axis
- Describe the role of APUD cells
- Describe the action of GI tract peptides and the stimuli for their release
- Describe the structure and function of the pineal gland and the role it plays in jet lag.

This chapter describes several tissues whose endocrine functions are still being realized:

- Gastrointestinal tract – secretes many hormones that regulate digestive function. Some act locally as mediators, some travel through the blood to act on distant organs
- Pineal gland – secretes melatonin, which regulates circadian rhythms.

ENDOCRINE CELLS IN THE GASTROINTESTINAL TRACT

Enteroendocrine cells are the product of one of the four stem-cell lineages that exist within intestinal epithelium and are considered to be part of the 'diffuse endocrine system'. They secrete a variety of peptides, in different combinations, in response to stimuli reflecting nutrient consumption and utilization (e.g. intestinal distension or chemical stimuli) both locally in the intestine and systemically. They potentiate or inhibit the release and action of each other. The main peptides will be considered individually below but the role of these peptides in concert is just beginning to emerge and this complex system may have a significant role to play in the treatment of obesity and diabetes in the future.

Some GI tract peptides, e.g. vasoactive intestinal polypeptide (VIP), cholecystokinin (CCK), gastrin, ghrelin and pancreatic polypeptides (PP), also act as neurotransmitters in the CNS and the neurons that innervate the GI tract (called the enteric nervous system). The following functions are regulated in the CNS by these peptide neurotransmitters:

- Biological rhythms – VIP
- Orexigenic (stimulate appetite) – ghrelin
- Anorexigenic (reduce appetite) – CCK, glucagon-like peptide-1 (GLP-1), oxyntomodulin (OXM), peptide tyrosine-tyrosine (PYY) and PP

- Adiposity signals – leptin and adiponectin
- Growth – somatostatin.

Together, these hormones and the vagus nerve constitute the 'gut–brain axis'. This intricate system relays information to the hypothalamus and brainstem about energy homeostasis in the GI tract. The 'gut–brain axis' serves a number of functions:

- Regulates food intake and appetite
- Regulates glucose and fat metabolism
- Regulates the secretion and sensitivity of GI tract hormones.

THE APUD CONCEPT

APUD cells are a group of endocrine cells that secrete small peptide hormones in many tissues throughout the body. The name 'APUD' (amine precursor uptake and decarboxylation) reflects the conversion of actively absorbed amine precursors into amino acids, which are used to make peptide hormones. These cells are linked by three features:

- Appearance under an electron microscope (e.g. neurosecretory granules)
- Biochemical pathway for amine or peptide hormone synthesis
- Embryological origin is from neural crest cells, which migrate to foregut and other locations.

They are also called neuroendocrine cells, due to their secretion of both neurotransmitters and 'hormones'. The following cells are examples of APUD cells:

- Islets of Langerhans cells which secrete insulin and glucagon
- Enteroendocrine cells (see below)
- Parafollicular cells which secrete calcitonin; they are found in the thyroid gland

- Juxtaglomerular complex that secretes renin; found in kidneys
- Neuroendocrine cells of the respiratory tract which secrete serotonin and calcitonin.

GASTROINTESTINAL TRACT PEPTIDES

The major peptides secreted by the GI tract are described below. Figs 6.1 and 6.2 show the location of GI tract peptide release and the major actions of four GI tract hormones. The actions of other peptides are shown in Fig. 6.3.

Delivery

GI tract peptides reach their target cells via two means:

- Endocrine – via blood
- Paracrine – act locally to affect nearby cells.

Some peptides have both endocrine and paracrine functions, e.g. somatostatin.

Gastrin

Gastrin is predominantly secreted by G cells in the antrum of the stomach after a meal. It is secreted in response to:

- Peptides or amino acids in the stomach
- Vagal stimulation (i.e. parasympathetic)
- Stomach distension
- Gastrin releasing peptide.

It acts to increase protein breakdown, specifically by:

- Stimulating enterochromaffin-like cells to secrete histamine. This acts on histamine-2 receptors (H_2) of parietal cells in the stomach to promote the release of hydrochloric acid and intrinsic factor
- Stimulating the release of hydrochloric acid directly through its action on the CCK receptors of parietal cells
- Stimulating parietal cell maturation and growth of the mucosa
- Stimulating chief cells to secrete pepsinogen
- Stimulating pancreatic hormone secretion

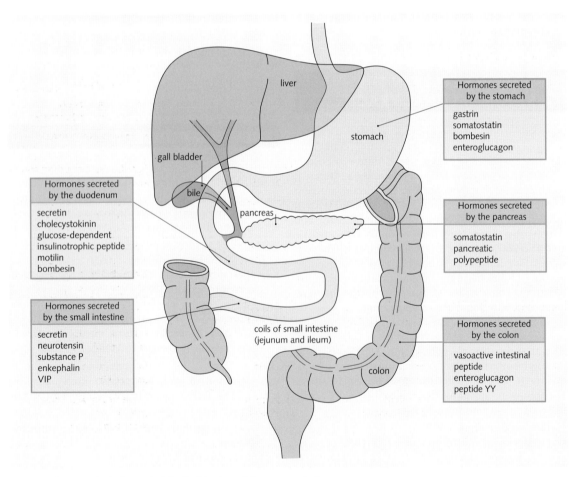

Fig. 6.1   Sites at which the gastrointestinal tract peptides are secreted.

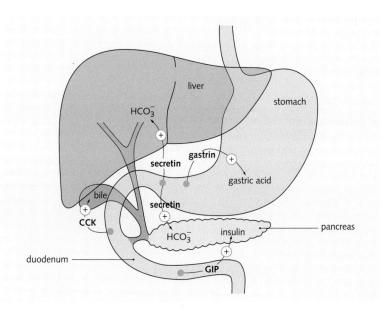

Fig. 6.2 Major actions of four gastrointestinal tract hormones. (CCK, cholecystokinin; GIP, glucose-dependent insulinotrophic peptide.)

Fig. 6.3 The sites of secretion, stimuli for secretion and actions of the minor gut peptides

Gut peptide	Site of secretion	Stimulus for secretion	Action of peptide
Enteroglucagon	A cells in the stomach and L cells in the colon	Presence of glucose and fat in the stomach	Reduces gastric acid secretion and gut motility
Bombesin	P cells in the stomach and duodenum	Fasting	Stimulates gastrin release
Motilin	EC cells in the duodenum	Absence of food in the duodenum	Speeds gastric emptying and stimulates colonic motility
Vasoactive intestinal polypeptide (VIP)	D1 cells and neurons in the small intestine and colon	Gut distension	Stimulates local gut secretion, motility and blood flow
Peptide YY (related to pancreatic polypeptide)	PYY cells of the colon	Presence of intestinal fat	Inhibits gastric motility and acid secretion (peptide YY is elevated in coeliac disease and cystic fibrosis)
Substance P	Enteric neurons in the small intestine	Cholecystokinin (CCK), 5-hydroxytryptamine (5-HT)	Stimulates gut motility, secretion and immune response; may have a role in inflammatory bowel disease
Enkephalin	Enteric neurons in the small intestine	Unknown	Inhibits gut motility and secretion
Neurotensin	N cells of the small intestine	Presence of intestinal fat	Stimulates local gut motility, secretion and immune response

- Promoting gastric motility
- Relaxing the pyloric and ileocecal sphincters.

Patients presenting with recurrent peptic ulcers, especially if there is a family history of endocrine cancers, should be investigated for Zollinger–Ellison syndrome. These patients have gastrin-producing pancreatic adenomas or islet hyperplasia, which causes excessive release of gastrin, over-stimulation of parietal cells, acidification of stomach contents and destruction and ulceration of the stomach mucosa.

Secretin

Secretin is secreted by the S cells of the duodenum and the small intestine in response to low pH in the duodenum and other luminal contents, including ethanol and products of protein metabolism. It neutralizes gastric acid by:

- Stimulating pancreatic secretion of fluid and bicarbonate ions (HCO_3^-)
- Inhibiting acid secretion from the parietal cells in the stomach.

Cholecystokinin

CCK is secreted by I cells in the duodenum and jejunum in response to fatty acids, lipids and certain amino acids. It is also found in the brain. It primarily increases the breakdown of fat by:

- Stimulating pancreatic enzyme and fluid secretion
- Stimulating gallbladder contraction and release of bile into the duodenum
- Potentiating the actions of secretin
- Causing some bicarbonate ion release from the pancreas
- Delaying gastric emptying
- Producing a sensation of satiety (fullness), causing a decrease in appetite.

Leptin and insulin

Both leptin and insulin act as long-term adiposity signals, regulating body weight. Leptin is produced predominantly by white adipose tissue in direct proportion to the amount of body fat present. Leptin therefore communicates the status of energy stores to the hypothamalus. Its actions include:

- Increasing satiety, which reduces appetite. This decreases food intake. This is brought about by actions on the hypothalamus
- Controlling energy expenditure
- Enhancing the effects of short-term satiety signals, e.g. CCK, GLP-1.

Ghrelin

This is a peptide secreted by P/D1 cells in the fundus of the stomach that:

- Stimulates appetite
- Stimulates growth hormone release from the anterior pituitary
- Decreases insulin secretion
- Stimulates gastric motility, gastric emptying and acid secretion.

Ghrelin levels rise before meals, stimulating appetite through its action on the hypothalamus. Levels drop after meals. Apart from the short-term effects, ghrelin may also contribute to long-term regulation of weight. This may have clinical implications in the future.

Adiponectin

Adiponectin is a collagen-like protein hormone secreted by adipose tissue. Plasma levels are inversely proportional to weight. It exhibits the following actions:

- Anti-inflammatory and anti-atherogenic effects. It prevents the formation of atherosclerotic plaques
- Anti-diabetic effects. Promotes insulin sensitivity.

Low levels of adiponectin are found in patients with excess abdominal and visceral fat. This is associated with a number of conditions:

- Obesity
- Type 2 diabetes
- Dyslipidaemia
- Hypertension
- Atherosclerosis
- Metabolic syndrome.

The further elucidation of the pathophysiological role of adiponectin in these conditions may yield therapeutic applications for their treatment in the future.

Glucagon-like peptide-1

Glucagon-like peptide-1 (GLP-1) is secreted by L cells in the ileum of the small intestine in response to nutrient ingestion. It has a number of actions:

- Enhances insulin release after oral glucose ingestion
- Suppresses glucagon release
- Delays gastric emptying and acid secretion
- May improve insulin sensitivity and restore β-cell mass in the pancreas
- Promotes satiety in the brain.

Unlike insulin, GLP-1 causes a decrease in weight. Due to its insulinotrophic effect, GLP-1 agonists have been developed to treat type 2 diabetes mellitus. Examples include exenatide and liraglutide.

Dipeptidyl peptidase-4 inhibitors

GLP-1 is rapidly degraded by the enzyme dipeptidyl peptidase-4 (DPP-4). This has somewhat limited the development of GLP-1 analogues. By blocking the action of DPP-4, the breakdown of endogenous GLP-1 is prevented, thereby prolonging its action. Examples include sitagliptin and vildagliptin. These are used to treat type 2 diabetes.

Glucose-dependent insulinotrophic peptide

Glucose-dependent insulinotrophic peptide (GIP), also called gastric inhibitory peptide, is secreted by the enteroendocrine K cells of the duodenum and jejunum in response to fats and carbohydrates. It acts to:

- Stimulate insulin secretion
- Inhibit gastric acid production and gastric motility.

This may have therapeutic applications for type 2 diabetes in the future.

Somatostatin

Somatostatin is secreted mainly by the δ cells of the islets of Langerhans in the pancreas but also by D cells in the stomach and duodenum. It is also secreted by the hypothalamus where it is called growth-hormone-inhibiting hormone (GHIH), and it inhibits the release of growth hormone and TSH. In the intestine, secretion is stimulated by:

- Low pH and amino acids in the stomach
- High blood glucose
- CCK
- Gastrin.

Somatostatin acts to slow down digestion by:

- Inhibiting secretion of gastrin, insulin and glucagon
- Inhibiting secretion of pancreatic enzymes and bile
- Inhibiting release of GIP, VIP and CCK
- Reducing gastric motility
- Increasing fluid absorption.

Synthetic somatostatin is used in the treatment of neuroendocrine tumours and acromegaly.

Pancreatic polypeptide

Pancreatic polypeptide is secreted by the F cells of the islets of Langerhans in the pancreas in response to protein in the stomach or low blood glucose. Its actions remain unclear but it slows the absorption of food by:

- Inhibiting gall bladder contraction
- Inhibiting pancreatic enzyme secretion.

It may also play a role in the regulation of appetite and food intake, which could have implications for the treatment of obesity.

Insulin and glucagon

Insulin and glucagon are both peptides secreted by enteroendocrine cells in the pancreas. The important functions they perform are described in Chapter 5.

PINEAL GLAND

Structure

Macrostructure

The pineal gland coordinates circadian (daily) rhythms of dark–light (day–night) cycles by secreting the hormone melatonin. Darkness stimulates its release.

It is a small gland found at the posterior end of the corpus callosum, forming a section of the roof in the posterior wall of the third ventricle (Fig. 6.4).

The pineal gland begins to calcify after puberty, making it a useful midline marker in X-rays and computed tomography (CT) scans.

Microstructure

The pineal gland is composed of two main types of neural cell:

- Pinealocytes – specialized secretory neurons
- Glial support cells.

In keeping with all endocrine organs, it has a very rich blood supply that forms a network of capillaries

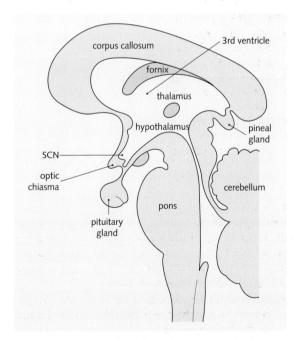

Fig. 6.4 Median section of the mid-brain and brainstem showing the anatomical location of the pineal gland and suprachiasmatic nucleus (SCN).

surrounded by the pinealocytes. It receives innervation from many parts of the brain, but the main connections are with the:

- Suprachiasmatic nucleus (SCN)
- Retina
- Sympathetic system
- Parasympathetic system.

Function

The pineal gland synthesizes and secretes the hormone melatonin (NB not melanin, the brown skin pigment). Melatonin is a modified form of the amino acid tryptophan, which is first converted to 5-HT then to melatonin.

There is evidence that reprogramming the pineal gland may help in the treatment of seasonal affective disorder.

Regulation

In the absence of light signals, circadian rhythms still exist but are not synchronized with the day–night cycle. The suprachiasmatic nucleus (SCN) in the hypothalamus serves as an 'intrinsic clock', which interacts with an external rhythm stimulus (or *Zeitgeber*), in this case light, to coordinate melatonin release with the external day–night cycle. This system allows the conversion of inhibitory light stimuli into a hormonal stimulus that can regulate:

- Day and night (circadian rhythm)
- Seasonal breeding rhythms (e.g. in deer, birds)
- Hibernation in animals.

Effects of melatonin

Melatonin has three main effects, which collectively serve to synchronize body physiology with environmental levels of light and darkness:

- It induces sleep (hypnotic effect)
- It resets the SCN
- It influences the hypothalamus, affecting behaviour.

Circadian rhythms influence almost every cell in the body. Hormones are secreted from the hypothalamus, pituitary gland and gonads with a circadian rhythm, e.g. secretion of corticotrophin-releasing hormone (CRH) and adrenocorticotrophic hormone (ACTH) peak early in the morning. These variations in hormone levels throughout the day are thought to be determined by the actions of the SCN and the pineal gland. The regulation and actions of melatonin are shown in Fig. 6.5.

Fig. 6.5 Regulation of melatonin and its actions.

Jet lag and melatonin treatment

The pineal gland has evolved to allow adaptation to changing day length (i.e. seasons). However, resetting of the SCN is best demonstrated by a jet flight in the following way:

- When a person leaves his or her home country the SCN and pineal gland are synchronized: at night, darkness and SCN activation stimulate melatonin production, inducing sleep.
- If the person flies across time zones, the SCN continues to oscillate in accordance with the previous time zone, which means that the timing of melatonin production (and, therefore, tiredness) does not change.
- At a rate of adjustment of a couple of hours a day, the SCN adapts to the new time zone.

Melatonin may also have therapeutic applications in the treatment of a range of other conditions, including:

- Alzheimer's disease
- Headaches
- Mood disorders.

Taking oral melatonin can shorten the period of jet lag. Melatonin should be taken at the times of darkness in the new time zone whilst on the plane and for several days at the destination. For shift work, the melatonin should be taken during the period of desired sleep. The SCN is reset more quickly and the body becomes resynchronized.

Endocrine control of fluid balance

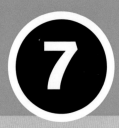

Fluid balance is important in maintaining appropriate perfusion of vital organs, in determining electrolyte concentrations and in meeting the body's demand for water. Humans have evolved to consume and store an excess of water at meal times, rather than being subject to constant thirst. Using this supply of water the body is able to adapt to demand by regulating renal water excretion. Changes in plasma concentration and plasma volume stimulate the release of hormones which regulate sodium and water reabsorption in the kidney. The variable reabsorption of sodium and water allows the body to be restored to equilibrium after fluid balance shifts outside the normal range. As blood pressure is affected by fluid balance, many of these hormones are also vasoactive. The main hormones involved in regulating fluid balance are:

- Antidiuretic hormone (ADH) – from the posterior pituitary gland (Fig. 7.1)
- Renin – from the kidney (Fig. 7.2)
- Aldosterone – from the adrenal cortex (Fig. 7.2).

An understanding of fluid balance is essential in medicine as it is a component in the management of many common conditions, e.g. heart failure and hypertension.

FLUID BALANCE

The importance of water

Water is needed for many normal physiological processes and is essential for all biochemical reactions. Water is contained in different compartments of the body, each containing a slightly different composition. There are two main fluid compartments in the body:

- Intracellular – makes up approx. 2/3 of total body water
- Extracellular – makes up approx. 1/3 of total body water.

Extracellular fluid (ECF) is further subdivided into blood plasma (makes up approx. ¼ of ECF) and interstitial fluid (makes up approx. ¾ of ECF). Interstitial fluid refers to fluid that bathes cells, CSF, intestinal fluid and fluid contained in joints.

This is the normal composition for an average 70-kg person; the amount of water in the body varies according to age, gender, and notably the amount of adipose tissue. As adipose tissue increases, total body water decreases.

All homeostatic mechanisms that regulate fluid balance respond to the composition of ECF. Receptors can only monitor plasma volume and osmotic concentration.

The importance of sodium

Fluid balance is intimately linked to sodium balance. Sodium ions are osmotically active (water follows sodium across cell membranes) and they are present in large quantities within the body. The normal plasma concentration of sodium ions is 135–145 mmol/L. In the kidney, variable water reabsorption is enabled by the kidney's ability to reabsorb variable amounts of sodium ions and, under certain conditions, by its ability to allow water to move more freely across cell membranes.

The importance of fluid volume

In addition to the maintenance of an adequate water supply, fluid balance, in particular, fluid volume is a key determinant of blood pressure. In order to ensure organs are adequately perfused the body is able to adapt to changes in fluid volume by adjusting:

- Cardiac output (i.e. stroke volume and rate)
- Peripheral resistance (i.e. vasodilatation or vasoconstriction).

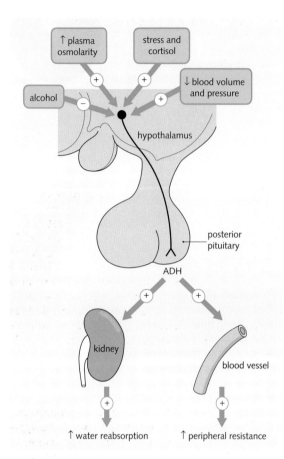

Fig. 7.1 Hormonal regulation of plasma osmolality by antidiuretic hormone (ADH).

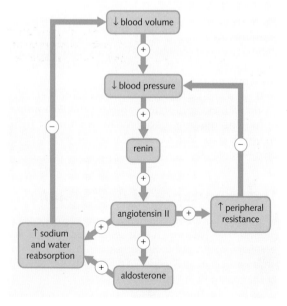

Fig. 7.2 Hormonal regulation of blood volume by renin, angiotensin II and aldosterone.

Determinants of fluid balance

Fluid balance involves the trade-off between fluid intake and fluid output, and the maintenance of the composition of the fluid.

Fluid intake

Water intake varies according to activity and climate, but around 2.5 L per day is required for normal functioning. Most of this is obtained by ingesting fluid. This comes in the form of food and drink and is often unconsciously acquired at meal times.

Fluid intake is determined by the sensation of thirst. Thirst is stimulated by the thirst centre in the hypothalamus. It contains osmoreceptors which monitor the osmolarity of the plasma. When plasma osmolarity increases or plasma volume decreases, thirst is the sensation which is produced and which causes us to consciously desire water.

Thirst can also be stimulated directly by angiotensin II and aldosterone which are closely linked to fluid balance in the kidney.

Fluid output

Water is mainly excreted by the kidney in the form of urine. Fluid is also excreted in faeces and sweat, and evaporates from the lungs and skin. The latter form brought about by evaporation is called 'insensible' fluid loss as we are unconsciously aware of the loss. Solutes are not lost in 'insensible' fluid, it is water only.

The total blood volume is about 5 L for a person of average weight and height. The kidneys filter this volume of blood about once every 5 minutes. Water and sodium are filtered into the kidney tubules by the glomeruli but most is reabsorbed back into the blood. Sodium ions are actively reabsorbed, while water passively follows the sodium by osmosis. Any sodium or water that is not reabsorbed is excreted in the urine.

Fluid balance can be regulated in the kidneys by altering two factors:

- Sodium reabsorption
- Permeability of the tubules to water.

Water is also lost by the processes shown in Fig. 7.3, but these losses are less significant than the actions of the kidney.

Fig. 7.3 Expected intake and output of water over a 24-hour period	
Water intake (mL)	**Water loss (mL)**
Drinking: 1500	Urine: 1500
Food: 500	Respiration: 400
Metabolism: 400	Skin evaporation: 400
	Faeces: 100
Total: 2400	Total: 2400

Factors that regulate fluid balance

Fluid balance is regulated by controlling the intake and excretion of water and sodium. Hormones regulate this balance by acting on:

- Thirst – detected and stimulated by the hypothalamus
- Volume and concentration of water excreted in the urine
- Peripheral resistance, which affects blood pressure.

There are three main hormones that regulate fluid balance; their sites and actions on the kidney nephron are shown in Fig. 7.4:

- Antidiuretic hormone (ADH; vasopressin) – regulates osmolarity of body fluids by conserving water. Also a potent vasoconstrictor
- Renin – stimulates angiotensin II synthesis and aldosterone release. Effects an increase in peripheral resistance in response to low arterial blood pressure, low plasma sodium levels or increased sympathetic activity
- Angiotensin II – conserves sodium and, as a result, water. Also a potent vasoconstrictor
- Aldosterone – conserves sodium and, as a result, water. Also a potent vasoconstrictor.

The following hormones, nerves and chemical factors are released in particular states and may modify the biological response to the former hormones, or act synergistically with them:

- Atrial natriuretic peptide (ANP) and brain natriuretic peptide (BNP)
- Renal sympathetic nerves and catecholamines
- Kinins
- Prostaglandins
- Dopamine.

HORMONES INVOLVED IN FLUID BALANCE

Antidiuretic hormone

This is the main hormone responsible for controlling volume of urine production. ADH acts on the kidney to conserve water. It increases the permeability of the distal tubule and collecting ducts to water, resulting in more water being reabsorbed and hence more concentrated urine production. ADH is also a potent vasoconstrictor. ADH regulates fluid balance by influencing the movement of water directly, not through sodium movement. Its main role is in maintaining water balance and not plasma volume. The regulation and actions of ADH are shown in Fig. 7.1.

Synthesis and secretion

ADH is a polypeptide hormone synthesized by neurosecretory cells in the supraoptic nucleus of the hypothalamus. It is transported along their axons to the posterior pituitary gland, where it is stored in vesicles. This process is described in more detail in Chapter 2.

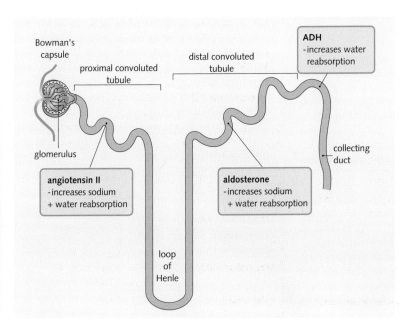

Fig. 7.4 Location and type of action by the three major hormones in the kidney nephron. (ADH, antidiuretic hormone.)

ADH is secreted by the posterior pituitary gland in response to stimuli which reflect a loss of intravascular water:

- High plasma osmolarity (concentrated blood). This is the more potent stimulus to ADH secretion
- Fall in blood pressure, which is detected by cardiac and large blood vessel baroreceptors.

ADH is rapidly degraded by the liver and kidney, enabling tight control of water balance.

Intracellular actions

ADH acts on G-protein-linked vasopressin receptors (V receptors) found on the cell surface of target cells. These target cells are found in two tissue types:

- Blood vessels – ADH acts on V_1 receptors causing smooth muscle contraction (i.e. vasoconstriction). Inositol triphosphate (IP_3) is the second messenger in this reaction
- Kidney – ADH acts on V_2 receptors in the kidney. This uses cAMP as a second messenger. In response to cAMP, aquaporins which are normally contained in cytoplasm vesicles fuse with the apical membrane and allow water to pass freely through the cell (the basolateral cell membrane is freely permeable to water). When cAMP is degraded, the aquaporin is removed from the apical cell membrane.

Effects

On the kidneys

ADH is secreted in response to high blood osmolarity. It increases the reabsorption of water at the kidney by increasing the permeability of the distal tubule and collecting duct. This water reabsorption is independent of sodium levels and therefore blood osmolarity can be decreased. Concentrated urine is produced.

On the blood vessels

ADH is also secreted in response to low blood volume. It causes arteriolar vasoconstriction, which increases peripheral resistance and raises blood pressure. This action is not usually involved in the regulation of blood pressure, but it is an important response to hypovolaemia in severe haemorrhage.

Deficiency and excess

ADH deficiency causes diabetes insipidus, in which excess dilute urine is produced, causing fluid dehydration, and high plasma osmolarity due to hypernatraemia.

ADH excess is called the 'syndrome of inappropriate antidiuretic hormone secretion and results in water retention'.

Both of these conditions are described in more detail in Chapter 2.

ADH secretion is inhibited by alcohol, causing large volumes of dilute urine to be excreted, resulting in dehydration the next morning.

The renin–angiotensin–aldosterone system

The renin–angiotensin II–aldosterone system acts to maintain normal blood volume and blood pressure of the ECF.

Renin is produced by the kidney in response to low tubular sodium content or low perfusion pressure, and causes the release of angiotensin II, which in turn causes secretion of aldosterone. Angiotensin II causes sodium reabsorption and consequently water reabsorption in the proximal convoluted tubule of the kidney. Angiotensin II also causes peripheral vasoconstriction, thereby increasing peripheral resistance, and raising blood pressure. The regulation and actions of angiotensin II are shown in Fig. 7.4.

Aldosterone causes the reabsorption of sodium and therefore water in the distal convoluted tubule and collecting ducts, and the secretion of potassium at the same sites.

Synthesis and secretion of renin

Renin is a small peptide enzyme secreted by the cells of the juxtaglomerular complex of the kidney. This complex is made of three cell types (Fig. 7.5):

- Juxtaglomerular cells – part of the afferent glomerular arteriole which secretes renin in response to a fall in sodium. Also responds to beta1 adrenergic activation which occurs when arterial blood pressure falls
- Macula densa – composed of chemoreceptor cells which monitor chloride ions in the distal convoluted tubule. This reflects the concentration of sodium ions in the tubule
- Extraglomerular mesangial cells – glomerular support cells that control blood flow in the afferent glomerular arteriole.

Renin release is also controlled by potassium levels, angiotensin II and ANP.

Renin release is stimulated by:

- Low blood pressure at the kidney
- Low tubular sodium levels
- Hypokalaemia.

Renin release is inhibited by:

- High blood pressure at the kidney
- High tubular sodium levels
- Hyperkalaemia.

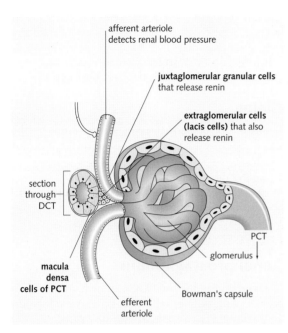

Fig. 7.5 Structure of the juxtaglomerular complex. (DCT, distal convoluted tubule, lying very close to the afferent and efferent arterioles; PCT, proximal convoluted tubule.)

Effects of renin

Renin is a proteolytic enzyme that acts on the plasma protein angiotensinogen which is synthesized by the liver. It cleaves this protein to form angiotensin I, which is then rapidly converted into angiotensin II by the action of angiotensin-converting enzyme (ACE) which is found in vascular beds, especially in the lungs. ACE inhibitors are a class of drug which are used to treat hypertension. Their effects are mediated by blocking the conversion of angiotensin I to angiotensin II by ACE.

Haemorrhage, dehydration, salt loss and renal artery stenosis all generate a stimulus for the juxtaglomerular cells to secrete renin. In most cases, this is a useful response to conserve water. However, in renal artery stenosis, the response is maladaptive and results in inappropriate sodium and water retention. Prostaglandins are involved in regulating the tone of the renal arterioles. Non-steroidal anti-inflammatory (NSAID) drugs, such as ibuprofen, inhibit prostaglandins, which can lead to renin release and resultant sodium and water retention.

Effects of angiotensin II

Angiotensin II has four important actions which serve to increase blood volume and pressure to appropriate levels:

- Stimulating aldosterone release from the adrenal cortex, which activates the pumps in the proximal tubule to increase sodium reabsorption, thereby increasing water reabsorption
- Peripheral vasoconstriction to raise blood pressure
- Stimulating sensation of thirst in the hypothalamus
- Inhibiting renin release (negative feedback).

Thus angiotensin II conserves sodium and water and raises blood pressure.

ACE inhibitors reduce blood volume and peripheral resistance by blocking the synthesis of angiotensin II by ACE. Both actions reduce blood pressure, so these drugs are useful in the treatment of hypertension and heart failure. ACE inhibitors also act on other substrates including kinins (e.g. bradykinin), which are thought to contribute to the hypotensive effect. Angiotensin II receptor blockers (ARBs) do not affect kinin levels and are also used to treat hypertension. They are often used when side effects from ACE inhibitors are intolerable.

A persistent dry cough is a common side effect of ACE inhibitors that is caused by the decreased degradation of bradykinin in the lungs. Bradykinin is usually broken down by ACE.

Aldosterone

Aldosterone is a mineralocorticoid synthesized by the zona glomerulosa cells of the adrenal cortex. The main stimulus for secretion is angiotensin II. Other factors that inhibit the synthesis of aldosterone include heparin, atrial natriuretic factor (ANF) and dopamine. Aldosterone causes the conservation of sodium and water. It regulates extracellular volume and potassium levels in the blood. See Chapter 4 for a complete description of aldosterone and the associated disorders. The regulation and actions of aldosterone are shown in Figs 7.2 and 7.4.

Aldosterone receptors are also found in the colon, illustrating its importance in regulating fluid levels.

Intracellular actions

Aldosterone acts on intracellular receptors in the distal convoluted tubule of the kidney. It causes sodium to be reabsorbed in exchange for potassium. Water follows this movement.

Effects

Aldosterone is secreted in response to high potassium levels or low blood volume through the actions of renin and angiotensin II. It acts to conserve sodium and water, thereby preventing its further release by negative feedback.

OTHER HORMONES INVOLVED IN THE REGULATION OF FLUID BALANCE

Natriuretic factors

Natriuresis is the excretion of large amounts of sodium in the urine. Diuresis is the production of large amounts of urine. Natriuretic factors have a diuretic effect, the opposite effect of ADH, angiotensin II and aldosterone. They increase sodium excretion, resulting in concomitant water excretion. This causes blood volume to decrease and blood pressure to drop. Natriuretic factors act as an 'escape mechanism' to prevent excessive water retention. Inappropriate natriuresis leads to a salt-losing syndrome entailing dehydration, hypotension and even sudden death.

Atrial natriuretic peptide (ANP) and brain natriuretic peptide (BNP)

ANP is a polypeptide hormone synthesized and stored in atrial myocytes and released in response to cardiac muscle distension due to high blood volume and fluid overload. ANP levels are a good indicator of hypervolaemic states, which occur in conditions such as congestive heart failure. A more sensitive diagnostic indicator of heart failure is BNP and NT-pro-BNP (which is a byproduct of BNP synthesis). These are synthesized by the ventricles (and also the brain, where they were discovered). Serum natriuretic peptides (especially BNP and NT-pro-BNP) should be measured in any patient with clinical signs and symptoms of heart failure. The serum level helps to guide management and dictates the severity of heart failure. Serum levels of BNP in particular correlate closely with prognosis in patients with congestive heart failure.

The main actions of natriuretic peptides are to stimulate natriuresis and diuresis by the kidney which lowers blood pressure. They do this by:

- Increasing the glomerular filtration rate. This is brought about by vasodilation of the afferent arteriole and vasoconstriction of the efferent arteriole of the glomerulus, increasing hydrostatic pressure in the capsule
- Decreasing sodium and water reabsorption by the kidneys
- Inhibiting renin, angiotensin II and aldosterone release.

Natriuretic peptides also cause dilation of veins, which reduces preload on the heart and therefore reduces cardiac output. They also cause arterial vasodilation, which decreases vascular resistance and therefore afterload on the heart; this reduces blood pressure.

Kinins

Kinins are potent vasoactive polypeptides formed in the blood vessels by the action of kallikrein on the precursor kininogen. They act in the kidney to:

- Inhibit the action of ADH
- Stimulate vasodilation in most vessels, but vasoconstriction of the pulmonary vasculature
- Stimulate prostaglandin synthesis
- Decrease sodium reabsorption.

Renal prostaglandins

Renal prostaglandins are locally acting lipid molecules synthesized by kidney cells. They act in the kidney to:

- Inhibit the action of ADH and aldosterone
- Stimulate vasodilatation in the kidney.

Dopamine

Dopamine is an amine synthesized in the proximal tubules. It acts in the kidney to:

- Inhibit tubular Na^+/K^+-ATPase and decrease sodium reabsorption
- Induce renal vasodilatation, thereby increasing renal bloodflow, glomerular filtration rate, natriuresis and diuresis.

DISORDERS OF FLUID BALANCE

A deficiency of water is called dehydration, which may or may not be accompanied by sodium deficiency. The causes and effects of dehydration are shown in Fig. 7.6.

An excess of water is called fluid retention, which may or may not be accompanied by an excess of sodium. The causes and effects of fluid retention are shown in Fig. 7.7.

Intravenous fluid replacement in patients otherwise unable to acquire fluids is essential. Normal daily fluid requirements (2400 mL) must be maintained and, in addition, extraordinary losses from haemorrhage, vomit or other causes must be restored. The principal fluid categories are crystalloids, colloids and blood products. Crystalloids include normal saline (0.9%), which is used to replace water and sodium but long-term use results in a drop in oncotic pressure and interstitial fluid accumulation (oedema).

Fig. 7.6 Causes and effects of dehydration

		Deficient sodium and water	Deficient water
Cause	Deficient input	Decreased ingestion, e.g. unconscious	Unable to find water, hypothalamic thirst disorder
	Excess output	Diarrhoea, vomiting, burns, haemorrhage, aldosterone deficiency	Diabetes insipidus and mellitus
Effect	Plasma osmolarity	No change	Raised
	Symptoms	Thirst, postural dizziness, weakness, collapse, headache, apathy, confusion, coma	
	Signs	Hypotension, tachycardia, slow capillary refill, reduced skin turgor, cool peripheries, sunken eyes, dry membranes, weight loss	

Fig. 7.7 Causes and effects of fluid retention

		Excess sodium and water	Excess water
Cause	Excess input	Excess fluid transfusion	Excess drinking, e.g. psychological or iatrogenic
	Deficient output	Cardiac, renal or hepatic failure	Renal hypoperfusion – cardiac, hepatic, renal causes or SIADH
Effect	Plasma osmolarity	No change, oedema	Decreased, no oedema
	Symptoms	Swelling of extremities or abdomen, dyspnoea, weight gain	Drowsiness, confusion, nausea, vomiting, anorexia, muscle weakness, headache, apathy, fits, coma
	Signs	Hypertension, raised JVP, displaced apex beat, ascites, peripheral pitting oedema	As above

JVP, jugular venous pressure.

Endocrine control of calcium homeostasis

8

● **Objectives**

By the end of this chapter you should be able to:
- Describe what happens when blood calcium levels rise and fall
- Describe the actions of the hormones responsible for maintaining calcium homeostasis
- Recall the aetiology, signs, symptoms, investigations and management of disorders of calcium homeostasis
- Define osteoporosis and osteopenia and recall the risk factors for developing osteoporosis
- Describe the principles of management of osteoporosis.

Hormones play an important role in the regulation of several mineral ions, notably calcium, phosphate and magnesium. Calcium is a cofactor for enzymatic reactions, a common intracellular signalling molecule and is essential for nerve conduction and skeletal, cardiac and smooth muscle contraction. It is also required for the release of neurotransmitters and both endocrine and exocrine hormones. Serum calcium levels must be tightly regulated to maintain these processes and prevent complications such as cardiac arrest. Hormones serve to maintain calcium homeostasis through their actions on the uptake of calcium in the intestines, release of calcium from the bone and excretion of calcium through the kidneys.

Blood calcium levels are regulated by three hormones (Fig. 8.1):

- Parathyroid hormone (PTH) – raises blood calcium levels
- Calcitonin – reduces blood calcium by increasing excretion of calcium
- Vitamin D_3 and its metabolite calcitriol – raise calcium intake from the gastrointestinal tract.

Blood calcium levels in the extracellular fluid (ECF) are kept within a very narrow range to maintain normal physiological processes. The two main hormones responsible for this are PTH and calcitonin which have opposing actions. They act on the free, ionized calcium in the blood. Calcium-sensing receptors on the parathyroid cells monitor serum calcium and release PTH in response to falling serum calcium levels. PTH has three target organs: the intestine, bone and kidneys. These effector organs act to increase serum calcium in response to PTH. An excess or deficiency of this hormone can cause hyper- and hypocalcaemia, respectively.

Important words:
Hyperparathyroidism: an excess of parathyroid hormone
Osteoclast: a cell that breaks down bone, releasing calcium
Osteoblast: a cell that lays down bone using calcium
Reabsorption: when substances are reclaimed from the kidney tubule after being filtered out of the blood.

THE ROLE OF CALCIUM

Calcium is a mineral obtained from the diet and excreted by the kidneys. Ninety-nine per cent of the total body calcium is in bone. The remaining 1% can be exchanged freely between plasma and the extracellular and intracellular compartments.

Calcium is essential for:

- Bone mineralization, acting in concert with phosphate ions (PO_4^-)
- Skeletal, cardiac and smooth muscle contraction
- All processes that involve exocytosis, including synaptic transmission and hormone release
- Enzymatic reactions
- Intracellular signalling.

The processes requiring calcium are described in Fig. 8.2.

Forty per cent of serum calcium is bound to albumin, a further 10% is bound to other proteins and the rest is in an unbound ionized form. Unbound ionized calcium (Ca^{2+}) is physiologically active and is the only component of blood calcium under direct influence of calcium-controlling hormones. It is the ionized

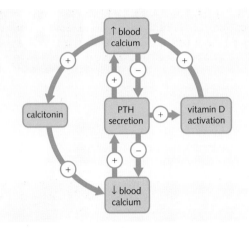

Fig. 8.1 Hormonal regulation of blood calcium by parathyroid hormone (PTH), vitamin D and calcitonin.

calcium which is most important. Normal levels are 1.0–1.25 mmol/L.

The amount of ionized calcium is affected by:

- Blood pH – calcium binding is reduced by low pH (acidosis) and increased by high pH (alkalosis). This increases and decreases free ionized calcium, respectively.

MECHANISMS INVOLVED IN CALCIUM HOMEOSTASIS

Calcium intake

The recommended daily allowance (RDA) of calcium is 1 g for normal adults, 1.2 g for pregnant women. If an individual is effectively maintaining the calcium balance, only 20% of the dietary calcium is absorbed. Absorption is influenced by:

- Diet – lactose in milk increases absorption; phytic acid in brown bread, tannins and caffeine in tea decrease absorption
- Age – absorption is increased in the young and decreased in the elderly
- Hormones – vitamin D increases absorption
- Pregnancy and lactation – both increase absorption.

Calcium balance

Calcium balance is calculated as absorbed calcium minus excreted calcium. This balance is affected by age and some diseases:

- Children usually have a positive calcium balance; this allows bones to grow.
- In adults, input and output should be the same.
- Postmenopausal women tend to have a negative calcium balance (i.e. calcium is lost).

Calcium in the blood

Calcium levels must be maintained within tight limits and the normal range of total serum calcium is 2.12–2.65 mmol/L. Dietary intake is variable, so the body must be able to adapt to increased or reduced plasma calcium. Calcium regulation involves the loss or gain of calcium via three tissues: kidneys, intestines and bones.

The movements and distribution of calcium in the body are shown in Fig. 8.3. The movements are regulated by the three hormones discussed below.

Fig. 8.2 Processes that require calcium	
System	**Role of calcium**
Bone formation	Calcium is a vital mineral component of bone; it makes the bone strong and rigid
Blood clotting	Many clotting factors are activated by calcium
Muscle contraction	Calcium binds to troponin, which allows myosin to bind to actin
Intracellular signalling	Calcium regulates the activity of a number of intracellular proteins in response to the second messenger IP_3
Nervous system	Calcium is essential for membrane potential and depolarization; synapses use calcium to release neurotransmitters
Endocrine system	All processes that involve exocytosis (e.g. hormone secretion) require calcium
Cardiovascular system	Calcium regulates the membrane potential and contraction of muscle cells

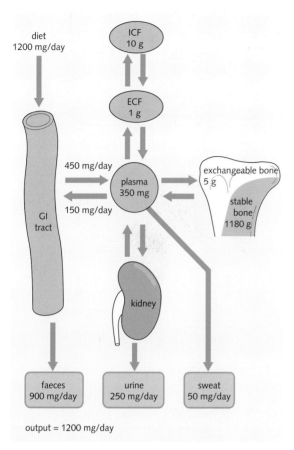

Fig. 8.3 Normal distribution and movements of calcium in the body. (ECF, extracellular fluid; GI, gastrointestinal; ICF, intracellular fluid.)

> Bone structures are dynamic and bone is constantly being broken down and remodelled.

Forty per cent of plasma calcium is bound to albumin. Diseases that lower plasma albumin (e.g. cirrhosis or myeloma) can increase unbound (i.e. active) calcium levels, causing symptoms and signs of hypercalcaemia. When measuring plasma calcium levels, it is total blood calcium that is measured. Albumin levels must be taken into account to calculate unbound, corrected calcium levels.

HORMONES INVOLVED IN CALCIUM HOMEOSTASIS

Three hormones regulate calcium levels in the blood and tissues:

- Parathyroid hormone from the parathyroid gland
- Vitamin D (cholecalciferol) from the diet and skin
- Calcitonin from the thyroid gland.

Their effects are summarized in Figs 8.1 and 8.4.

Parathyroid hormone and the parathyroid glands

PTH is synthesized by the chief cells in the parathyroid glands. The four small glands are located on the posterior surface of the lateral lobes of the thyroid gland. The principal effects of PTH are to increase serum calcium and reduce serum phosphate.

PTH is released in response to falling blood calcium levels. Its actions are to raise calcium levels back to their normal physiological concentration. Once blood calcium levels are restored to within the normal range, PTH production is inhibited.

Increases in blood phosphate also stimulate PTH release indirectly by binding to ionized calcium and thereby reducing its 'concentration'.

Parathyroid glands

Blood supply, nerves and lymphatics

The parathyroid glands are four oval-shaped structures about 5 mm across; they are embedded in the thyroid capsule behind both lateral lobes. These glands are described as superior and inferior pairs. The number of parathyroid glands often varies between two and six

Fig. 8.4 Summary of the actions of parathyroid hormone (PTH), calcitonin and vitamin D on calcium regulation

	PTH	Vitamin D	Calcitonin
Secreted/activated in response to:	Low blood calcium	PTH	High blood calcium
Kidneys	Calcium reabsorbed; vitamin D activated	Calcium reabsorbed	Calcium excreted
Bones	Calcium released	Calcium trapped	Calcium trapped
Intestines	Negligible	Calcium absorbed	Negligible

and the location of the inferior pair differs widely. They are supplied by branches of the inferior thyroid artery.

Microstructure

There are three cell types in the parathyroid glands:

- Chief cells – synthesize parathyroid hormone (PTH)
- Oxyphil cells – are inactive endocrinologically, but they can form Hürthle cell carcinomas
- Adipocytes – contain fat and their numbers also increase with age.

Development

The parathyroid glands are endodermal structures that develop from the pharyngeal pouches. The inferior parathyroid glands are formed by the dorsal portion of the third pouch, while the dorsal portion of the fourth pouch forms the superior parathyroid glands.

Parathyroid hormone

Synthesis and receptors

PTH is a polypeptide hormone composed of 84 amino acids. Falling plasma ionized calcium and low plasma ionized calcium trigger the release of PTH from vesicles, up-regulation of PTH transcription and, under conditions of chronic hypocalcaemia, can stimulate the chief cells to proliferate. Under normal conditions, calcium inhibits PTH release at near-maximal capacity. The system is therefore well-suited to adapt to a sudden fall more than a sudden rise in plasma calcium. Chief cells also possess a circadian rhythm, releasing PTH in a pulsatile manner.

PTH acts via G-protein-linked receptors on the cell surface. These receptors are found on osteoblasts, renal tubule cells and cells in the intestinal epithelium. The receptors use cyclic AMP (cAMP) as a second messenger to regulate the phosphorylation of intracellular proteins. These proteins are either activated or deactivated as a result; this brings about the effects of PTH.

Actions

PTH is the most important regulator of blood calcium levels. The actions of PTH on calcium regulation are shown in Fig. 8.5.

On the kidneys

PTH has three major effects:

- Increase of calcium ion reabsorption by stimulating active uptake in the distal convoluted tubule and thick ascending limb
- Increase of phosphate ion excretion by inhibiting uptake in the proximal and distal convoluted tubules. This causes more ionized calcium to be free in the circulation
- Stimulation of 1α-hydroxylase, an enzyme that activates vitamin D.

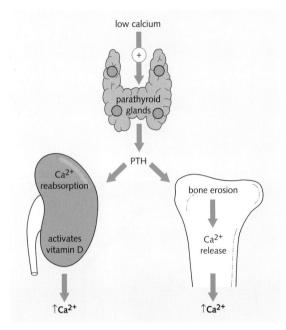

Fig. 8.5 Actions of parathyroid hormone (PTH) on the kidney and bone.

On the bones

PTH causes the release of calcium and phosphate from the bone. PTH stimulates osteoblast proliferation and differentiation and therefore increases bone production. PTH receptors are not found on osteoclasts but these cells are stimulated indirectly by factors released by the activated osteoblasts. Up-regulation of osteoclastic activity causes increased bone breakdown. The resultant increase in bone turnover can have different effects on net bone mass but always results in increased serum calcium. The actions are:

- Direct inhibition of osteoblast collagen synthesis
- Indirect stimulation of osteoclast bone erosion
- Increased collagenase synthesis to erode the bone
- Increased hydrogen ion release to create an acidic environment to enhance bone erosion.

On the intestines

PTH may have a direct action on calcium absorption in the upper small intestine, but this is unproven. The major effects are indirect, by stimulating 1α-hydroxylase. This causes the production of calcitriol, which promotes calcium and phosphate reabsorption in the intestine.

Although PTH causes increased mobilization of phosphate, due to the PTH-mediated excretion of phosphate in the kidney, the overall effect is to reduce serum phosphate levels.

Vitamin D

Vitamin D_3 (cholecalciferol) is absorbed by the small intestine as part of the diet (e.g. dairy food) or is synthesized from cholesterol in the skin. Vitamin D_3 synthesis requires ultraviolet B (UVB) light, usually derived from the sun. It is then converted into calcitriol. Calcitriol is the biologically active form of vitamin D and is a major determinant of intestinal calcium and phosphate reabsorption.

Activation

Human vitamin D is an inactive steroid called cholecalciferol (or vitamin D_3); this fat-soluble steroid is stored in adipose tissue. Two reactions must take place in different organs to activate vitamin D; they are shown in Fig. 8.6.

The activated vitamin D (1,25-dihydroxycholecalciferol) molecule is shown in Fig. 8.7. It can be inactivated by 24-hydroxylase found in the kidney. This enzyme catalyses the formation of 1,24,25-trihydroxycholecalciferol, which is rapidly excreted.

All forms of vitamin D are transported in the blood by a specific plasma protein (transcalciferin). Vitamin D is fat-soluble, so it can cross cell membranes. It acts via specific intracellular receptors that are found in the same locations as PTH receptors.

Actions

The actions of vitamin D on calcium regulation are shown in Fig. 8.8.

On the intestines

The main action of vitamin D (calcitriol) is stimulation of active calcium and phosphate absorption in the duodenum and jejunum. The exact mechanism is unclear; however, it is thought that Ca^{2+}-ATPase is up-regulated and transcription of a calcium-binding protein (calbindin) is stimulated by vitamin D (calcitriol). This makes the intestine more permeable to calcium. This action on the intestines takes a long time to produce an effect, so it does not raise calcium levels immediately.

On the kidney

Activated vitamin D has three effects:

- Increase of calcium reabsorption in the proximal and distal convoluted tubule
- Increase of phosphate reabsorption in the proximal convoluted tubule
- Inhibition of 1α-hydroxylase activity. This is a form of negative feedback.

On the bones

Vitamin D affects bone remodelling by modulating calcium levels and by directly stimulating osteoblast activity (and indirectly osteoclasts). This brings about the conditions of high calcium and phosphate optimum for bone mineralization. Disorders of vitamin D absorption or activation can result in inadequate mineralization of bones (rickets in children or osteomalacia in adults). If this is due to kidney disease, it is called renal osteodystrophy (discussed later).

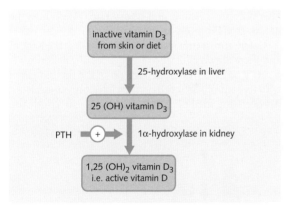

Fig. 8.6 Activation of vitamin D. (25(OH) vitamin D_3, 25-hydroxyvitamin D_3; 1,25(OH)$_2$ vitamin D_3, 1,25-dihydroxyvitamin D_3.)

Calcitonin

Calcitonin is secreted by the parafollicular cells (C cells) in the thyroid gland. The development and anatomy of this gland is described in Chapter 3. Calcitonin is secreted as blood calcium rises, and it lowers calcium levels. It has actions antagonist to PTH. It is not essential to life, but it acts to fine-tune blood calcium levels.

Synthesis and receptors

Calcitonin is a polypeptide hormone that is formed by the breakdown of a larger prohormone. Calcitonin is stored in secretory vesicles, from which it is released when blood calcium levels rise. Rising calcium is detected by the same calcium-sensing receptor which is present on parathyroid cells.

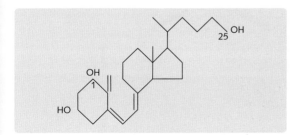

Fig. 8.7 Structure of 1,25-dihydroxyvitamin D_3, the active form of vitamin D.

Fig. 8.8 Actions of vitamin D on the gastrointestinal tract, bone (PTH, parathyroid hormone) and kidney.

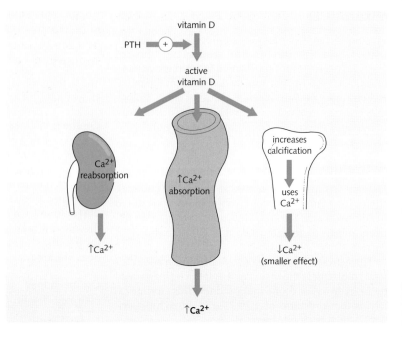

Calcitonin acts on G-protein-coupled receptors that release cAMP to bring about cellular effects.

Actions

The actions of calcitonin on calcium regulation are shown in Fig. 8.9.

On the kidney

Calcitonin inhibits the reabsorption of calcium and phosphate. These ions are excreted as a result.

On the bones

Calcitonin acts primarily on osteoclasts in the bone. It inhibits these cells to prevent all stages of bone erosion. This prevents calcium and phosphate release into the blood, so their levels are lowered.

Calcitonin is not essential for calcium regulation, and there are no clinical consequences of calcitonin deficiency or excess. Neither removal of the thyroid gland with its parafollicular cells at thyroidectomy nor calcitonin-secreting medullary cell malignancy affect calcium

Fig. 8.9 Actions of calcitonin on the kidney and bone.

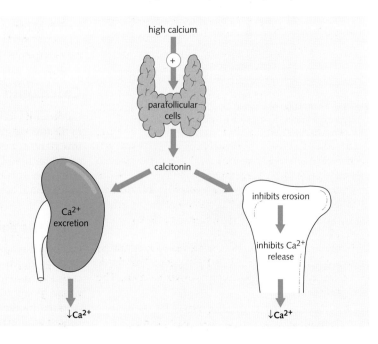

balance significantly. Calcitonin is used therapeutically to reduce pain associated with vertebral fractures and to treat Paget's disease (a condition of excessive bone resorption).

> Never give the antibiotic tetracycline to young children, as it binds to calcium in their teeth, making them yellow. In adults, milk should not be used to swallow tablets of tetracycline.

Phosphate

Calcium and phosphate are regulated by similar processes and together they constitute 65% of the weight of bone. They form hydroxyapatite crystals, which mineralize the bone and give it strength. Phosphate is also an essential component of nucleic acids, phospholipid membranes, ATP and signalling molecules. PTH-induced bone resorption causes the release of phosphate. However, phosphate lowers ionized calcium levels and therefore antagonizes the calcium-raising ability of PTH. This potential antagonism is overcome by PTH concomitantly exerting a strong phosphaturic action, thereby keeping phosphate low whilst trying to raise serum calcium.

DISORDERS OF CALCIUM REGULATION

Since PTH is the most important hormone in calcium homeostasis, disorders of this system are grouped according to their effect on PTH release. The two groups are:

- Hyperparathyroidism (excess of PTH)
- Hypoparathyroidism (deficiency of PTH).

Primary hyperparathyroidism

Primary hyperparathyroidism is excessive PTH release. All the actions of PTH raise calcium levels, so hypercalcaemia (excess blood calcium) results. Hypercalcaemia and excess PTH cause the symptoms shown in Fig. 8.10. Prolonged hyperparathyroidism causes bone demineralization and softening, called osteomalacia in adults and rickets in children. The symptoms and signs of these diseases are shown in Fig. 8.11.

Primary hyperparathyroidism is a relatively common endocrine disorder (about 1 in 1000 people), and it is especially common in postmenopausal women. The main causes are:

- Parathyroid gland adenoma (80%)
- Diffuse parathyroid gland hyperplasia (15%).

Neoplastic chief cells are not inhibited by high calcium, and consequently PTH secretion is unregulated. Malignant tumours of the parathyroid gland are very rare, but they can be associated with other endocrine tumours in multiple endocrine neoplasia (MEN) syndromes. These are discussed in Chapter 10.

> When clerking a patient with suspected hypercalcaemia, remember: 'Bones, stones, abdominal groans and psychic moans'.

Diagnosis and treatment

Primary hyperparathyroidism is usually detected on routine testing and is suspected if a patient has:

- Unexpected bone weakness
- Hypercalcaemia symptoms and signs
- Hypercalcaemia on a blood test with low phosphate levels
- Dehydration
- Severe thirst.

It is investigated by:

- Blood test – measuring fasting serum calcium and phosphate. This will show raised serum calcium and reduced serum phosphate
- Measuring blood PTH (increased)
- Measuring renal function. This is often normal but should be measured as a baseline
- Radiography may show subperiosteal bone resorption of the phalanges
- Radioisotope scanning or ultrasound of the parathyroid glands to detect adenomas
- Elevated serum alkaline phosphatase may be seen in parathyroid bone disease
- 24-hour urinary calcium should be measured in young patients who present with a moderate increase in serum calcium and PTH to exclude familial hypocalciuric hypercalcaemia.

Additionally, an abdominal X-ray could be performed to detect nephrocalcinosis or renal calculi due to hypercalcaemia.

Medication should be reviewed. Common medications (e.g. lithium and thiazide diuretics) can cause hypercalcaemia.

There are three treatment options:

- Restrict dietary calcium and vitamin D, and encourage adequate hydration
- Drug treatment (e.g. calcitonin, bisphosphonates, cinacalcet in certain patients). This is reserved for patients who do not fulfil the criteria for surgery
- Surgical removal of the parathyroid gland(s). Some indications for surgery include patients under 50 and patients with a serum calcium >3.00 mmol/L.

Fig. 8.10 Symptoms and signs of hypercalcaemia.

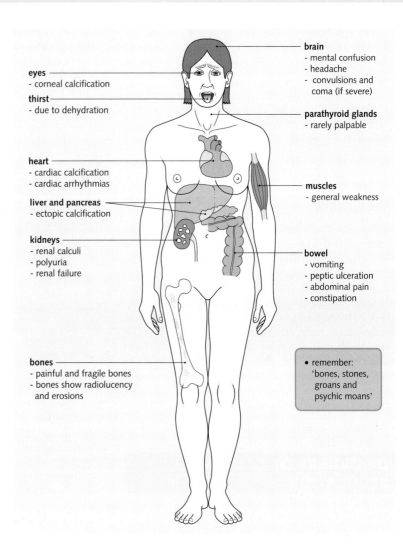

eyes
- corneal calcification

thirst
- due to dehydration

heart
- cardiac calcification
- cardiac arrhythmias

liver and pancreas
- ectopic calcification

kidneys
- renal calculi
- polyuria
- renal failure

bones
- painful and fragile bones
- bones show radiolucency and erosions

brain
- mental confusion
- headache
- convulsions and coma (if severe)

parathyroid glands
- rarely palpable

muscles
- general weakness

bowel
- vomiting
- peptic ulceration
- abdominal pain
- constipation

- remember: 'bones, stones, groans and psychic moans'

Fig. 8.11 Signs and symptoms caused by rickets and osteomalacia

Rickets (childhood)	Osteomalacia (adulthood)
'Knock-knees' or 'bow-legs' caused by bending of the long bones	Bone pain
Chest deformities, back deformities (e.g. kyphosis) and protruding forehead	Bones appear 'thin' on X-ray, with localized lucencies (called Looser's zones)
Features of hypocalcaemia	Fractures (common in the neck of the femur)
	Features of hypocalcaemia (e.g. proximal myopathy causes waddling gait)

A contraindication for parathyroid surgery is familial hypocalciuric hypercalcaemia.

Common complications of parathyroid surgery include:

- Hypocalcaemia
- Recurrent laryngeal nerve injury
- Bleeding and haematoma formation.

Secondary hyperparathyroidism

Many diseases can cause hypocalcaemia (e.g. chronic renal failure), which stimulates PTH as a compensatory response. If hypocalcaemia is prolonged the glands enlarge by hyperplasia to secrete excess PTH. This is called secondary hyperparathyroidism. It is characterized by raised PTH with normal or low serum calcium.

Causes of secondary hyperparathyroidism

Hypocalcaemia can be caused by:

- Chronic renal failure
- Vitamin D deficiency or malabsorption.

In chronic renal failure, the kidneys fail to reabsorb calcium. Renal osteodystrophy is a complication of chronic kidney disease characterized by:

- Secondary hyperparathyroidism
- Osteomalacia
- Vitamin D deficiency.

It is caused by:

- Impaired 1α-hydroxylase activity in the kidney. This leads to reduced vitamin D activation and less calcium reabsorption. This increases PTH production.
- Impaired phosphate clearance by the kidney. Hyperphosphataemia reduces the amount of ionized calcium, leading to increased PTH production.
- PTH-induced reabsorption of calcium from bone, leading to bone marrow fibrosis and cyst formation. This can be identified radiologically and is called osteitis fibrosa cystica.

Vitamin D deficiency can occur if the diet is deficient in vitamin D or the skin does not receive adequate sunlight (e.g. people who spend excessive amounts of time indoors or extensive skin covering) of the right wavelength to produce vitamin D (UVB). Deficiency of activated vitamin D causes hypocalcaemia as a result of impaired calcium absorption in the intestines. Reduced intestinal absorption and reduced mobility occur in the elderly as a normal process, so they are at a higher risk of developing vitamin D deficiency. Clinically there is a normal amount of bone but it does not mineralize fully – osteomalacia in adults, rickets in children.

Treatment aims to correct the cause. This may include:

- Dietary modification and/or phosphate binders
- Vitamin D analogues
- Modification of dialysis
- Cinacalcet (calcimimetic). This is not recommended for patients with end-stage renal disease on dialysis.

Tertiary hyperparathyroidism

Tertiary hyperparathyroidism is a complication of secondary hyperparathyroidism and is seen in patients with renal failure. If secondary hyperparathyroidism persists, the level of calcium required to inhibit PTH production by the parathyroid glands is reset to a higher level. This causes autonomous parathyroid gland activity and hypercalcaemia. Parathyroidectomy is often indicated at this stage.

Familial hypocalciuric hypercalcaemia

This is a rare genetic condition which is characterized by raised renal reabsorption of calcium in the presence of hypercalcaemia. It is caused by a mutation of the calcium-sensing receptor in the parathyroid glands, resulting in deficient binding, and this raises the set-point for calcium homeostasis. Diagnosis depends on family history and a reduced calcium/creatinine clearance ratio in blood and urine samples. No treatment is indicated and parathyroid surgery does not solve the problem.

Hypoparathyroidism

Hypoparathyroidism is the deficiency of PTH resulting in hypocalcaemia. It causes the usual symptoms of hypocalcaemia (see Fig. 8.12) but without osteomalacia. The main causes are listed below:

- Complication of thyroid or parathyroid surgery
- Congenital deficiency – DiGeorge syndrome
- Idiopathic hypoparathyroidism – an autoimmune disorder
- Pseudohypoparathyroidism – congenital PTH resistance.

Investigations reveal reduced serum calcium and increased serum phosphate.

Pseudohypoparathyroidism is the result of resistance to PTH. Patients have raised PTH with the symptoms of hypoparathyroidism.

Hypocalcaemia may cause carpopedal spasm, which can be elicited by occluding the brachial artery with a blood-pressure cuff for over 3 minutes (Trousseau's sign). Hypocalcaemia can also be demonstrated clinically by the twitching of the ipsilateral facial muscles in response to tapping on the facial nerve (Chvostek's sign). If hypocalcaemia is suspected on

Fig. 8.12 Symptoms and signs of hypocalcaemia.

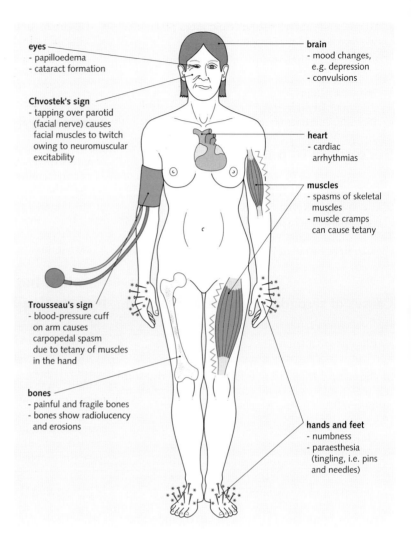

eyes
- papilloedema
- cataract formation

brain
- mood changes, e.g. depression
- convulsions

Chvostek's sign
- tapping over parotid (facial nerve) causes facial muscles to twitch owing to neuromuscular excitability

heart
- cardiac arrhythmias

muscles
- spasms of skeletal muscles
- muscle cramps can cause tetany

Trousseau's sign
- blood-pressure cuff on arm causes carpopedal spasm due to tetany of muscles in the hand

bones
- painful and fragile bones
- bones show radiolucency and erosions

hands and feet
- numbness
- paraesthesia (tingling, i.e. pins and needles)

clinical examination the common causes can be recalled using the mnemonic HARVARD: **H**ypoparathyroidism (also hyperphosphataemia and hypomagnesaemia), **A**cute pancreatitis, **R**enal failure, **V**itamin D$_3$ deficiency, **A**lkalosis, **R**habdomyolysis, **D**rugs (e.g. bisphosphonates).

Osteoporosis

Osteoporosis is a disease characterized by low bone mass and deterioration of bone sufficient to cause bone fragility and an increased risk of fracture. It is defined as a bone mineral density (BMD) 2.5 standard deviations (or less) below the mean BMD for young, healthy adults at peak bone mass. Osteopenia is defined as 1–2.5 standard deviations below normal BMD.

It is caused by increased osteoclast activity and breakdown of bone and decreased bone formation by osteoblasts. This causes loss of bone mass; however, adequate bone mineralization still occurs.

Since new bone is poorly formed, microfractures cannot be repaired, so the bones become thin and brittle.

Loss of bone is a normal part of the ageing process; however, women are at a greater risk due to the loss of oestrogen production after menopause. There are a number of other risk factors for osteoporosis including:

- Family history of osteoporotic fractures
- Rheumatoid arthritis
- Long-term corticosteroid use
- Alcohol intake of >4 units per day and smoking
- Vitamin D deficiency and hyperparathyroidism in the elderly.

Osteroporosis is responsible for approximately 180 000 fractures in England and Wales every year.

Management comprises prevention and pharmacological treatment. Strategies include:

- Calcium and vitamin D supplements
- Exercise
- Physiotherapy assessment for risk of falls
- Smoking cessation and avoiding excessive alcohol
- Bisphosphonates (e.g. alendronate)
- Strontium ranelate and raloxifene (second line)
- Teriparatide-recombinant human PTH (third line)
- Calcitonin

- Hormone replacement therapy (HRT) for post-menopausal women, particularly younger women.

The risk factors and pharmacological treatment of osteoporosis sections are adapted, with permission, from National Institute for Health and Clinical Excellence (2008) 'TA 161 Alendronate, etidronate, risedronate, raloxifene, strontium ranelate and teriparatide for the secondary prevention of osteoporotic fragility fractures in postmenopausal women – Quick reference guide'. London: NICE. Available from http://www.nice.org.uk/.

Endocrine control of growth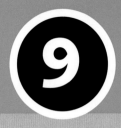

9

Objectives

After reading this chapter, you should be able to:
- Describe the roles, actions and regulation of growth hormone and IGFs
- Name other factors affecting growth
- Name four peptide growth factors, the tissues that secrete them, and where they affect
- Understand how to determine height and mean parental height
- Understand the principal diagnosis and management of growth disorders
- Describe the main changes that occur in the body during puberty.

Growth hormone (GH) is a pituitary hormone that can act directly on tissues throughout the body; however, its main effects are mediated by insulin-like growth factors (IGFs). These are secreted from the liver in response to GH. In this way, growth follows the conventional pattern of starting in the hypothalamus (described in Chapter 2).

Growth is a process that takes place at many levels. It can be defined as an increase in:

- Anabolism (e.g. protein synthesis)
- Cell size and number
- Cell mutation and maintenance
- Organ size
- Body size or weight.

Acting through IGFs, GH stimulates all the processes listed above. By promoting anabolic processes, the cell increases in size. This promotes cell division and maturation, causing the organ to grow. The cellular actions of GH begin at birth and continue throughout life, though the level of action varies. The fastest rate of growth is in the fetus and neonate; however, a growth spurt also occurs during puberty.

The growth of the body is limited by the epiphyses (growth plates) at the ends of the long bones. GH stimulates these plates to grow, causing bones to lengthen and body height to increase. It also stimulates fusion of these growth plates preventing further growth.

> Important words:
> **Anabolism**: the process of building large molecules from smaller ones
> **Epiphysis**: the end of a long bone (*plural* epiphyses)
> **Epiphyseal growth plate**: an area of cartilage between the epiphysis and shaft of the bone that proliferates during childhood, resulting in elongation of the bone

> **Growth factor**: any chemical that stimulates cellular growth
> **Cell maturation**: when a cell differentiates to reach its final form

DIRECT CONTROL OF GROWTH

Growth hormone (GH)

GH (also called somatotrophin) is a polypeptide that is secreted by the somatotroph cells in the anterior pituitary gland. Like many pituitary hormones, it is synthesized as a precursor molecule (pre-progrowth hormone). Two cleavages release the active hormone. For more information about the anterior pituitary, see Chapter 2.

Regulation of secretion

GH secretion is regulated by two hypothalamus releasing factors:

- Growth-hormone releasing hormone (GHRH)
- Somatostatin (also called growth-hormone inhibiting hormone or GHIH).

GHRH is released in a pulsatile manner, especially during deep sleep or hypoglycaemia, and GH release follows this pattern. Secretion of GH from the anterior pituitary gland is also regulated by the negative feedback of IGF-1 and other growth factors (Fig. 9.1).

Effects

GH promotes the growth and maintenance of most cells. It exerts most of its effects by:

- Stimulating the uptake of amino acids
- Stimulating the synthesis of proteins.

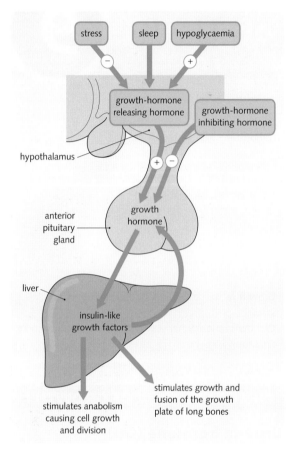

Fig. 9.1 Hormonal regulation of growth hormone.

GH exerts most of its effects via IGFs. GH promotes their synthesis, mainly in the liver but also in other tissues.

GH is transported in the blood bound to GH-binding protein. It acts via G-protein and Janus kinase (JAK) receptors on the cell surface of the target cells.

Insulin-like growth factors

Insulin-like growth factors (IGFs or somatomedins) are polypeptide hormones that exist in two forms: IGF-1 and IGF-2. They resemble insulin in structure and they act via similar receptors. IGF-1 is more important as a stimulator of growth. It is transported in the blood by a number of IGF-binding proteins.

Metabolic actions

Both IGF hormones have some insulin-like actions, e.g. increasing amino acid uptake and protein synthesis. However, they also oppose the actions of insulin on glucose by preventing glucose uptake and causing glycogen breakdown to raise blood glucose.

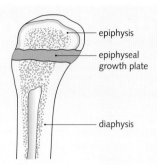

Fig. 9.2 The regions of a growing bone.

Growth actions

The increase in protein synthesis caused by the metabolic effects of IGF hormones causes cells to grow. This stimulates cell division and maturation, causing organs and soft tissues to enlarge.

The growth of the long bones depends on the state of the epiphyseal growth plate. This is a layer of chondrocytes (cartilage cells) located between the end (epiphysis) and shaft (diaphysis) of the bone (Fig. 9.2). Before puberty, IGFs stimulate these chondrocytes to grow, divide and mature into osteocytes (bone cells), allowing the bone to lengthen whilst maintaining a population of chondrocytes in the plate for further growth. During puberty, IGFs and sex steroids stimulate the chondrocytes within the plate to mature into osteocytes so that the epiphysis and diaphysis become fused together. The bone is no longer able to lengthen with further IGF stimulation so final adult height is reached.

Other growth factors

Growth in specific tissues is also stimulated by a number of growth factors, many of which are small peptides that act in a paracrine (local) manner. Their relationship to GH is not known. The actions and secretion of several such peptides are described in Fig. 9.3.

INDIRECT CONTROL OF HORMONES

Many factors apart from GH control growth, including:

- Genetics – tall parents often have tall children
- Adequate nutrition – however, excess nutrition does not increase height
- Health – chronic disease affects height
- Other hormones.

Fig. 9.3 The secretion of growth factors and their effects

Growth factor	Mode of delivery	Action on growth and development	Method and control of secretion
Nerve growth factor (NGF)	Paracrine	Induces neuron growth and helps to guide growing sympathetic nerves to organs they will innervate (may also act on the brain and aid memory retention)	Secreted by cells in path of growing axon; regulation of secretion not yet understood
Epidermal growth factor (EGF)	Paracrine and endocrine	Promotes cell proliferation in the epidermis, maturation of lung epithelium and skin keratinization	Secreted by many cell types, i.e. not only epidermal cells (EGF is also found in breast milk); regulation of secretion not yet understood
Transforming growth factors (TGF-α, TGF-β)	Paracrine	Stimulate growth of fibroblast cells; TGF-α acts similarly to EGF; TGF-β especially affects chondrocytes, osteoblasts and osteoclasts	Secreted by most cell types but especially platelets and cells in placenta and bone; regulation of secretion not yet understood
Fibroblast growth factor (FGF)	Paracrine	Mitogenic effect in several cell types; may induce angiogenesis (formation of new blood vessels), which is essential for growth and wound healing	Secreted by most cell types; regulation of secretion not yet understood
Platelet-derived growth factor (PDGF)	Paracrine	Potent cell-growth promoter; chemotactic factor (involved in inflammatory response)	Secreted by activated blood platelets during blood vessel injury
Erythropoietin	Endocrine	Stimulates the production of erythrocyte precursor cells	Secreted by the kidney in response to falling tissue oxygen concentration
Interleukins (IL) (33 known)	Autocrine and paracrine	IL-1 stimulates B-cell proliferation and helper T cells to produce IL-2; IL-2 autoactivates helper T cells and activates cytotoxic T cells	IL-1 is secreted by activated macrophages; IL-2 is secreted by activated helper T cells

Other hormones

Growth problems can be caused by the abnormal secretion of a number of hormones, including:

- Insulin
- Antidiuretic hormone (ADH)
- Parathyroid hormone and vitamin D
- Cortisol
- Sex steroids.

Thyroid hormones

Thyroid hormones, described in Chapter 3, stimulate cell metabolism, promoting cell growth and division, especially in the skeleton and developing central nervous system (CNS). Thyroid hormones also stimulate GH secretion from the pituitary.

Cortisol is described in Chapter 4; it inhibits pituitary GH secretion, so chronic ill health or stress can suppress growth.

Normal growth can only occur if both the hormone milieu and the nutritional supply of proteins are suitable.

Fetal growth

In the fetus, a hormone called placental lactogen is secreted from the placenta. It stimulates fetal cartilage development and acts in a similar manner to prolactin on the maternal mammary glands.

Thyroid hormones are essential for the development of the skeleton and CNS. A deficiency in the fetus or neonate results in cretinism.

Puberty

Sexual maturation and the pubertal growth spurt are described later in this chapter.

DETERMINATION OF HEIGHT

A person's final height is determined simply by the rate and duration of growth.

During puberty, the epiphyseal growing plates at the end of the long bones begin to fuse. This fusion prevents further growth and, therefore, further height gain.

Complete fusion occurs between 18 and 20 years of age in males, and earlier in females.

Fusion of the epiphyseal plates is stimulated primarily by GH and sex steroids; however, thyroid hormone also promotes this effect. A simple increase in GH during puberty is not sufficient to increase final height since bones simply mature faster and stop growing.

Only the bones that grow in this manner are prevented from responding to further GH. The jaw and skull can continue to grow past puberty; this effect is seen in GH excess. Ultimately, height is determined by multiple genetic factors.

Short stature, defined as a height less than the third centile, is associated with poor academic achievement and anxiety. Growth rates less than the 25th centile will result in a child dropping down centiles on a growth chart. Short stature can be primary, secondary or idiopathic. Primary disorders reflect an intrinsic bone defect and include achondroplasia and some causes of intrauterine growth retardation. Secondary disorders occur in the presence of other factors that limit bone growth. Malnutrition, chronic disease and endocrine disorders, such as Cushing's, can also be secondary causes. Idiopathic short stature is the most common cause of short stature and is a variant of normal.

DISORDERS OF GROWTH

Excess of growth hormone

Excess GH prior to epiphyseal fusion causes gigantism, proportional abnormal growth. Since the epiphyses also fuse at an earlier age, the child may have an unremarkable height in adulthood. Diabetes is very common in this group because of the opposing actions of insulin and GH on blood glucose.

An excess of GH is slightly more common in adults, where it manifests as acromegaly (prevalence approximately 60 per million). The signs and symptoms are shown in Fig. 9.4. The long bones can no longer lengthen, so there is no increase in height. However, the soft tissues and other bones can still grow, causing the distinctive features of this condition (Fig. 9.5). Acromegaly is a serious condition, associated with an increase in mortality from cardiovascular disease, respiratory disease and malignancy. A therapeutic reduction in plasma GH is effective in reducing this excess mortality.

GH-secretion pituitary adenomas are the most common cause of acromegaly. These adenomas can cause other symptoms by compressing surrounding structures (e.g. pituitary stalk compression). Assessment of acromegaly should therefore include demonstration of excess GH, localization of the tumour, global assessment of anterior pituitary function and assessment of metabolic and structural complications.

Diagnosis

Excess GH can be diagnosed by high IGF-1 levels, but the best test is to measure GH levels following an oral glucose tolerance test. GH levels should fall with the rise in glucose. Computed tomography (CT) or magnetic resonance imaging (MRI) scans can be used to confirm the presence of a functional pituitary adenoma.

Treatment

The mainstay of treatment is surgical removal of the tumour. At 3 months post-op, a day curve of GH levels is measured (4–5 samples, aiming for a mean GH >5 mU/L) or a repeat oral glucose tolerance test (OGTT), measure IGF-1, and do pituitary function tests to rule out hypopituitarism.

Additional treatments may be needed if surgery is unsuccessful. These include somatostatin/GHIH analogues, recombinant GH analogue (acts as a GH receptor antagonist) and radiotherapy.

Deficiency of growth hormone

The deficiency of GH in children is called dwarfism. It is detected by short stature along with either:

- Dropping between growth chart centiles (i.e. not following the expected course)
- Being significantly shorter than mean parental height (MPH).

The most common cause of dwarfism is a deficiency of GHRH from the hypothalamus; craniopharyngiomas can also be responsible. See Chapter 2 for more details.

Diagnosis and treatment

GH deficiency is diagnosed using a stimulation test. Impaired GH rise is seen after sleep, hypoglycaemia induced by IV insulin (used less often because of risks) or an arginine stimulation test. The treatment for GH deficiency is subcutaneous injections of recombinant human growth hormone (rhGH) before sleep each night.

Genetic short stature

Children can be short as a consequence of genetics without pathological correlates. These children have short parents and they start growing below the 5th centile but at a normal rate with a normal age of pubertal onset. Mean parental height (MPH) is the average of the parents' heights plus 7 cm in males or

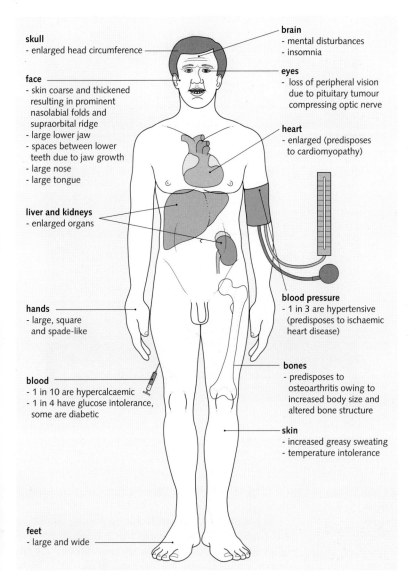

Fig. 9.4 The symptoms and signs of acromegaly.

skull
- enlarged head circumference

face
- skin coarse and thickened resulting in prominent nasolabial folds and supraorbital ridge
- large lower jaw
- spaces between lower teeth due to jaw growth
- large nose
- large tongue

liver and kidneys
- enlarged organs

hands
- large, square and spade-like

blood
- 1 in 10 are hypercalcaemic
- 1 in 4 have glucose intolerance, some are diabetic

feet
- large and wide

brain
- mental disturbances
- insomnia

eyes
- loss of peripheral vision due to pituitary tumour compressing optic nerve

heart
- enlarged (predisposes to cardiomyopathy)

blood pressure
- 1 in 3 are hypertensive (predisposes to ischaemic heart disease)

bones
- predisposes to osteoarthritis owing to increased body size and altered bone structure

skin
- increased greasy sweating
- temperature intolerance

minus 7 cm in females. Constitutional delay in growth and maturation involves delayed puberty and a delayed pubertal growth spurt, but the normal adult height is attained.

PUBERTY

Puberty is when the sexually immature child becomes a sexually fertile adult. Prepuberty girls and boys develop pubic and axillary hair. This prepubertal phase is the result of adrenache (Chapter 3). Puberty starts with the reactivation of gonadotrophin (LH and FSH) release

after the dormancy of childhood. The age of pubertal onset varies widely between individuals (females 8–13 years; males 9–14 years). Puberty is characterized by a number of processes:

- Pubertal growth spurt
- Development of secondary sexual characteristics
- Achievement of fertility
- Psychological and social development.

Gonadarche and the initiation of puberty

From an endocrine perspective, puberty is marked by the onset of pulsatile gonadotrophin release from the anterior pituitary gland during the night.

Fig. 9.5 X-ray of the skull showing acromegaly

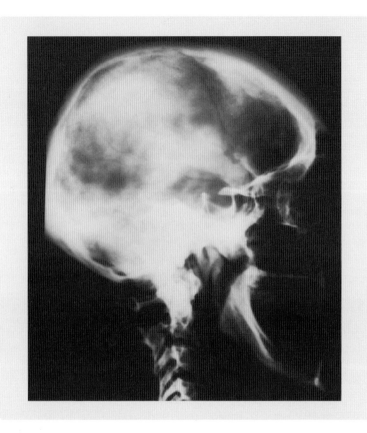

Gonadotrophins stimulate the production of sex steroids (i.e. testosterone and oestrogen) from the gonads; the activation of the gonads is gonadarche.

The onset of puberty is not fully understood; however, the CNS integrates a number of signals. According to the gonadostat hypothesis, a reduction in hypothalamic sensitivity to the negative feedback of the sex steroids causes the hypothalamus to secrete higher levels of gonadotrophin-releasing hormone (GnRH) in a pulsatile manner. Secretion of growth hormone (GH), thyroid-stimulating hormone (TSH) and adrenocorticotrophic hormone (ACTH) is also increased. Other evidence favours the central maturation of the CNS and its common final communication pathways between the hypothalamus GnRH neurons and the pituitary.

Body weight and puberty

In the last few decades the onset of puberty has occurred at an increasingly young age. This change is often attributed to improved nutrition and rising body weight

of 47 kg is a better predictor of the start of periods than age.

In recent years, a possible mechanism for this effect has been found. The hormone leptin is secreted by the adipose tissue, and is a hormonal indicator of body fat: higher levels of leptin are present with increasing body fat. Leptin may be the trigger for GnRH activation. Puberty cannot begin without leptin, but evidence suggests that it is only one of a number of factors. The exact details of the causal relationship between a critical metabolic mass derived from lean body weight, body fat and total body water and the onset of puberty remains unclear.

The pubertal growth spurt

The earliest developmental event in puberty is an increase in growth velocity called the growth spurt. It occurs about 2 years earlier in females, giving a temporary height advantage. The initial rise in growth velocity is slight, so growth of the breasts or testes is usually noticed first.

The increase in growth is caused by increased GH and sex steroid secretion. Sex steroids also cause bone maturation. As the bones mature, the growing plates (epiphyses) fuse, preventing further growth. This fusion occurs 2 years earlier in females, giving males an extra 2 years of growth. This largely accounts for the increased height of adult males.

Puberty in the male

Puberty usually occurs between 9 and 14 years of age in boys; however, it is considered normal if it occurs between 9 and 16 years of age. Once the testes have developed, male pubertal changes are brought about by the secretion of androgens such as DHT and testosterone.

Testes development and early puberty

Growth of the testes from <2 mL to >4 mL is often the first sign of puberty noticed in boys around 12 years. The increase is mainly due to proliferation of the seminiferous tubules under the influence of FSH. LH stimulates the interstitial Leydig cells to secrete testosterone. The scrotum becomes larger, thicker and pigmented; pubic hair growth follows.

Spermatogenesis begins once the testes have enlarged and matured and is associated with a rise in serum inhibin B. Nocturnal emissions and daytime ejaculations are often around 13–14 years of age at stage 3 of Tanner's male genital staging, with fertile ejaculations around 15 years.

> **HINTS AND TIPS**
>
> Clinically, male puberty has begun when the testes reach 4 mL. This is measured with an orchidometer.

Penile development and late puberty

The penis begins to enlarge after the testes about the same time the growth spurt is noticed. The penis doubles in size during puberty to reach an average size of 9.5 cm flaccid or 13.2 cm erect.

> Klinefelter's syndrome (XXY) is associated with small testicles, abnormal spermatogenesis and infertility. The syndrome is also associated with delayed motor learning. Treatment is with testosterone. Women with Turner's syndrome lack part of the X chromosome (or a whole X chromosome) needed for normal ovarian

development and acquisition of normal secondary sexual characteristics. These women are often amenorrhoeic, infertile and have abnormal breast and pubic hair development. Treatment is with oestrogen to promote sexual development and growth hormone to encourage growth.

Facial and axillary hair growth usually starts at about 15 years of age. The sebaceous glands in the skin are also activated, often causing acne.

The breaking of the voice is also a late feature. The larynx, cricothyroid cartilage and laryngeal muscles enlarge to give an Adam's apple.

> **HINTS AND TIPS**
>
> Tanner's staging is used to assess puberty milestones and compare individuals. The stages are based on testis, scrotum and penile growth and pubic hair in males:
> Stage 1: height increases 5 cm per year, no pigmented pubic hair, testes volume <4 mL, no penis growth.
> Stage 2: height increases 5 cm per year, small amount of pigmented pubic hair, testes volume 4–6 mL, increased penis dimensions. Stage 3: height increases 7.5 cm per year, darker pubic hair, testes volume 8–10 mL, increased penis dimensions. Stage 4: height increases 10 cm per year, testes volume 14–16 mL, increased penis dimensions, adult pubic hair quality. Stage 5: adult pubic hair distribution, testes volume 18–25 mL, maximum height reached, mature penis size reached.
> Additional changes: axillary hair, increased muscle mass, voice breaks.

Puberty in the female

Puberty in females usually occurs between 8 and 13 years of age in girls; however, it is considered normal between 8 and 15 years of age. The changes caused by oestrogens and progesterone are shown in Fig. 9.6.

Breast development and early puberty

The development of breast buds is often the first sign of puberty noticed in girls. The breast then continues to grow under the influence of oestrogen while the ductal system develops; the number of lobules remains the same from infancy (Fig. 9.6). Pubic hair begins to grow about 6 months later.

Fig. 9.6 The changes caused by oestrogen and progesterone during female puberty

Oestrogen-mediated changes	Progesterone-mediated changes
Fat deposition and proliferation of the ductal system in the breasts, causing growth	Proliferation of the secretory lobules and acini in the breast
Growth of the vagina and maturation of the epithelium	Contribution to vaginal and uterine growth
Growth of the clitoris	Initiation of cyclical changes in endometrium and ovary

Menarche and late puberty

The uterus begins to enlarge after the development of pubic hair. The onset of menstruation (periods) is called menarche. The mean age of menarche is 13 years, making it a late feature of puberty. In the ovary, follicular development begins and the first ovulation occurs 10 months after the first menarche, on average, i.e. the early menstrual cycle are often anovulatory and infertile.

Tanner's stages and the female

In the female, the stages are based on breast and pubic hair development.

Breast development

Stage 1: preadolescent, only papillae are elevated. Stage 2: breast bud develops with papillae and breasts elevated. Stage 3: juvenile smooth stage with further growth of breasts and areolae. Stage 4: areolae and papillae project above the breasts. Stage 5: adult pattern with areolae on the same level as the rest of the breasts.

Pubic hair development

Stage 1: preadolescent, no pubic hair. Stage 2: sparse hair on labia majora. Stage 3: darker, coarser and curlier hair, spreads over pubis. Stage 4: adult-type pattern but covers smaller area. Stage 5: adult pattern.

Endocrine disorders of neoplastic origin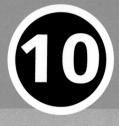

Objectives

By the end of this chapter you should be able to:
- Describe the theories of MEN tumour formation
- List the common tumours associated with each of the MEN syndromes
- Describe the theories behind ectopic hormone secretion
- List tumours that secrete hormones ectopically, along with the relevant tumour
- Understand carcinoid tumours and carcinoid syndrome.

Endocrine organs can undergo neoplastic change and non-endocrine organs can acquire an endocrine phenotype as a result of neoplastic change. When several different endocrine tumour types affect a single individual they are usually part of a multiple endocrine neoplasia (MEN) syndrome. These syndromes result when several endocrine disorders, share a common genetic basis. There are three patterns, referred to as MEN-I, MEN-IIa and MEN-IIb. These syndromes are rare, but they can cause tumours in young adults. They are usually inherited and genetic testing can be used to determine the risk in family members.

Other endocrine syndromes are caused when tissues outside the endocrine system give rise to 'ectopic' hormone-secreting tumours. These tumours can present with symptoms pertinent to the hormone that is being secreted.

MULTIPLE ENDOCRINE NEOPLASIA SYNDROMES

MEN syndromes are clusters of endocrine tumours that often occur in the same patient. The tumours are rare, usually aggressive and arise in multiple tissues; they occur earlier than single sporadic tumours. The underlying cause is probably genetic, since these syndromes are usually inherited in an autosomal dominant fashion although some cases are sporadic.

MEN syndromes are rare, but they may be life-threatening.

The following patterns of MEN have been described: MEN-I, MEN-IIa, MEN-IIb (Fig. 10.1) and FMTC.

MEN-I (Werner's syndrome)

The most common tumours are:
- Parathyroid hyperplasia – most common
- Pancreatic islet cell tumours/duodenal tumours
- Pituitary adenoma (secrete growth hormone, prolactin or ACTH).

The pancreatic islet cell tumours may secrete ectopic hormones (e.g. glucagonoma or insulinoma) and the duodenal tumours may secrete gastrin causing Zollinger–Ellison syndrome. Thirty per cent of the very rare Zollinger–Ellison tumours are caused by MEN-I.

MEN-1 is caused by loss-of-function of a tumour suppressor gene, the *MEN-I* gene, which produces a protein that regulates cell proliferation. Patients typically have a germline mutation in one allele and acquire somatic mutations in the other allele. MEN-II syndromes are caused by gain-of-function mutations in the *RET* proto-oncogene. The precise genetic location of this mutation determines the exact phenotype. If family members test positive for these mutations, they can be treated with prophylactic surgery.

Less commonly, MEN-I is associated with:
- Parathyroid adenoma
- Hyperplasia of thyroid parafollicular cells
- Adrenal cortical hyperplasia.

MEN-IIa (Sipple's syndrome)

The main tumours of the MEN-II syndrome are:
- Phaeochromocytoma (often bilateral)
- Medullary cell carcinoma of the thyroid (MTC, often multi-focal, age of onset <30).

Occasionally, parathyroid hyperplasia can develop.

Fig. 10.1 The principal tumours and hormones associated with the three MEN syndromes

Syndrome	Associated tumours	Hormones secreted
MEN-I	Parathyroid hyperplasia, pancreatic islet cell, pituitary adenomas	PTH, insulin, prolactin
MEN-IIa	Medullary carcinoma of the thyroid, phaeochromocytomas	Calcitonin, adrenaline
MEN-IIb	Medullary carcinoma of the thyroid, phaeochromocytomas, neuromas	Calcitonin, adrenaline

MEN, multiple endocrine neoplasia; PTH, parathyroid hormone.

MEN-IIb

The very rare MEN-IIb is sometimes called MEN-III. MEN-IIb patients get both phaeochromocytomas and MTC, although the MTC is usually more aggressive and is present before 5 years of age. Patients also have a marfanoid appearance (long axial bones). Two other types of tumour develop in the skin and submucosa throughout the body:

- Neuromas (tumours of neurons)
- Ganglioneuromas (tumours of neuronal ganglia).

Familial medullary thyroid carcinoma (FMTC)

Medullary thyroid cancer can also occur in a hereditary pattern without the other endocrine abnormalities. Seventy-five per cent of MTC is not familial. Calcitonin is a good plasma marker for following the progression of MTC.

ECTOPIC HORMONE SYNDROMES

Ectopic hormones

'Ectopic' means out of place. The term 'ectopic hormone' is used when a tissue secretes a hormone that it does not normally secrete. The hormone is released in an uncontrolled manner by a tumour (benign or malignant). The tumour can be:

- Endocrine tissue secreting unusual hormones
- Non-endocrine tissue secreting any hormone.

Symptoms are usually caused by the excess of the ectopic hormone while the tumour is still small. Examples of syndromes caused by ectopic hormone secretion are listed in Fig. 10.2.

Treatment

The tumours are treated in a similar manner to any symptomatic tumour, i.e.:

- Surgical removal
- Irradiation
- Chemotherapy.

Aetiology of ectopic hormones

The exact mechanism behind ectopic hormone release is not fully understood, and it may vary between tumours. There are two main theories:

- The tumour originates from cells that normally secrete small amounts of hormones, e.g. cells of the bronchial mucosa normally secrete adrenocorticotrophic hormone (ACTH) and anaplastic carcinoma of the lung secretes ectopic ACTH.
- Mutations associated with the transformation to neoplasia activate dormant genes, resulting in ectopic hormone production.

Types of ectopic hormone

Ectopic hormones are almost always peptide hormones because their synthesis requires expression of only a single gene. Steroid hormone synthesis requires the expression of a complicated series of enzymes.

The ectopic hormone is often not an exact version of a normal hormone, e.g. breast cancer cells secrete PTH-related peptide. This would fit the second theory of aetiology, since the normal processing enzymes may not be present.

CARCINOID TUMOURS

These are tumours of the APUD cells of the small intestine, most commonly affecting the appendix, terminal ileum and rectum. They can also occur in other locations in the GI tract, bronchus and the sexual organs.

Fig. 10.2 Examples of syndromes caused by ectopic hormone secretion

Syndrome	Hormone secreted by tumour cells	Tumour
Hypercalcaemia	PTH or PTH-like peptide	Squamous cell carcinoma of the lung, breast carcinoma
Hyponatraemia	ADH	Oat cell carcinoma of the bronchus, some intestinal tumours
Hypokalaemia (symptoms of Cushing's syndrome caused by ACTH excess take longer to develop)	ACTH and ACTH-like peptides	Oat cell carcinoma of the bronchus, medullary carcinoma of the thyroid, thymic carcinoma, islet cell tumours
Gynaecomastia	Human placental lactogen	Carcinoma of the bronchus, liver or kidney
Galactorrhoea	Prolactin	Carcinoma of the bronchus, hypernephroma
Polycythaemia	Erythropoietin	Hypernephroma, carcinoma of the uterus
Hypoglycaemia	Insulin (rare)	Hepatomas, large mesenchymal tumours
No syndrome	Calcitonin	Oat cell carcinoma of the lung

ACTH, adrenocorticotrophic hormone; ADH, antidiuretic hormone; PTH, parathyroid hormone.

Carcinoid tumours are normally asymptomatic until metastases occur, though the tumour may cause some symptoms as it grows. Some tumours in the appendix can cause appendicitis as they cause obstruction.

These tumours can also secrete a variety of hormones, including insulin, glucagon, ACTH (can cause Cushing's syndrome), thyroid and parathyroid hormones. Other secretions include serotonin, tachykinins, bradykinins, gastrin and prostaglandins. These tumours can appear with other neuroendocrine tumours or as part of MEN-I syndrome.

CARCINOID SYNDROME

This occurs in around 5% of patients with carcinoid tumours and indicates liver involvement. Typically patients will complain of flushing, especially in the face and neck (most likely a result of bradykinins), as well as recurrent periods of diarrhoea and abdominal pain. Patients can also develop cardiac complications due to serotonin-induced pulmonary fibrosis and tricuspid incompetence.

Diagnosis

Diagnosis involves looking for the secondary signs of the tumour itself, specifically ultrasound for liver metastases and 24-hour urine collection to measure the main metabolite of serotonin. This is called 5-hydroxyindoleacetic acid.

Treatment

The mainstay of treatment is surgery to remove the tumour.

Hormones of the reproductive system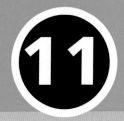

Objectives

After reading this chapter, you should:
- Know the relevant anatomy of both male and female genitalia
- Understand the hormones secreted by the different organs and their function
- Understand the hormonal changes in the body associated with pregnancy, labour and lactation.

The reproductive systems in both men and women are controlled in many ways by the endocrine system, as seen in puberty. The reproductive organs themselves produce hormones that can influence the rest of the body. This chapter focuses on the normal functions of these organs and the actions of the hormones they release.

The main functions of the female reproductive system are:

- Oogenesis and ovulation – production and release of oocytes (female gametes)
- Fertilization – allowing the sperm and oocyte to meet and fuse
- Pregnancy – providing a suitable environment for the fetus to grow
- Parturition – expelling the fetus with minimal trauma to the baby and mother
- Lactation – providing nutrition for the baby.

After menarche (the start of periods), the female body prepares for pregnancy every month until menopause. This process is regulated by four main hormones (Fig. 11.1):

- Follicle-stimulating hormone (FSH)
- Luteinizing hormone (LH)
- Oestrogen
- Progesterone.

The male reproductive system consists of the testes, prostate, seminal vesicles and the penis. Its principal functions are:

- Sperm production (spermatogenesis) and release
- Production of hormones involved in male reproduction and libido.

After puberty, the testes begin to produce sperm and they continue to do so until death. This process is regulated by four main hormones (Fig. 11.2):

- Follicle-stimulating hormone (FSH)
- Luteinizing hormone (LH)
- Testosterone
- Inhibin B.

Further details on development and disorders of the reproductive systems are covered in other textbooks (*Crash Course Renal and Urinary Systems* and *Crash Course Obstetrics and Gynaecology*). Polycystic ovary syndrome is a disease of the female reproductive system and is covered in this chapter.

THE FEMALE REPRODUCTIVE SYSTEM

Anatomy

The female reproductive system consists of six main components (Fig. 11.3):

- Ovaries – produce oocytes and female sex steroids (e.g. oestrogens)
- Uterine (fallopian) tubes – connect the ovaries to the uterus; they are the normal site of fertilization
- Uterus – supports the implantation and development of the fetus
- Vagina – normal site for the deposition of sperm
- Vulva – the structures surrounding the introitus (external orifice of the vagina)
- Breasts – produce milk.

The blood supply, lymphatics and innervation of the female reproductive organs are shown in Fig. 11.4.

Hormones

Ovarian sex steroids

The ovaries produce a number of steroid hormones in response to gonadotrophins from the anterior pituitary. The main hormones produced are:

- Oestrogens, e.g. oestradiol
- Progestogens, e.g. progesterone
- Androgens, e.g. androstenedione.

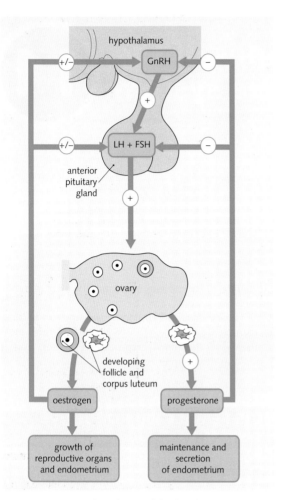

Fig. 11.1 Hormonal regulation of the female reproductive system. (FSH, follicle-stimulating hormone; GnRH, gonadotrophin-releasing hormone; LH, luteinizing hormone.)

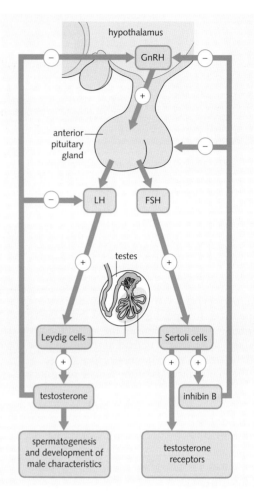

Fig. 11.2 Hormonal regulation of the male reproductive system. (FSH, follicle-stimulating hormone; GnRH, gonadotrophin-releasing hormone; LH, luteinizing hormone.)

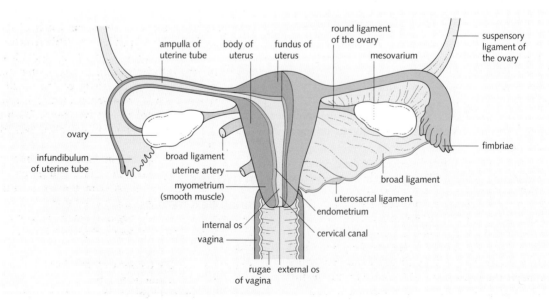

Fig. 11.3 Structure of the ovaries, uterine (fallopian) tubes and uterus.

Fig. 11.4 Blood supply, lymphatics and innervation of the female reproductive organs

Organ	Arterial supply	Venous drainage	Innervation	Lymphatic drainage
Ovaries	The ovarian arteries from the aorta via the suspensory ligaments	Forms the pampiniform plexus that drains into the ovarian veins in the suspensory ligaments	Autonomic nerves via the suspensory ligaments	Para-aortic lymph nodes
Uterine tubes	Uterine and ovarian arteries	Uterine and ovarian veins	Uterovaginal plexus and suspensory ligaments	Iliac, sacral and aortic lymph nodes
Uterus	Uterine arteries, branches of the internal iliac arteries	Forms a plexus in the broad ligament that drains into the uterine veins	Uterovaginal plexus in the broad ligament	Iliac, sacral, aortic (and inguinal) lymph nodes
Vagina	Uterine arteries from the internal iliac arteries	Vaginal venous plexus that drains into the internal iliac veins	Uterovaginal plexus in the broad ligament	Iliac and superficial inguinal lymph nodes
External genitalia	Pudendal arteries	Pudendal veins	Pudendal and ilioinguinal nerves, S2–S4	Superficial inguinal lymph nodes
Breasts	Internal thoracic, lateral thoracic and intercostal arteries	Axillary and internal thoracic veins	Intercostal nerves, mainly T4	Axillary and parasternal lymph nodes and the contralateral breast

Oestrogens

Oestrogens are secreted at the start of the menstrual cycle in response to LH and FSH. Their synthesis takes place in the developing ovarian follicle (Fig. 11.5), requiring both the thecal and granulosa cells. The theca interna secretes androgens in response to LH. LH activates the enzyme that converts cholesterol to pregnenolone (i.e. the first step in steroid production); however, the thecal cells lack the aromatase enzyme necessary to convert androgens to oestrogens.

The majority of androgens cross the basement membrane into the granulosa cells. FSH activates the aromatase enzyme produced by granulosa cells, allowing the thecal androgens to be converted to oestrogens (mainly oestradiol-17β). The process of oestrogen synthesis is shown in Fig. 11.6. After ovulation, oestrogens are produced by the corpus luteum formed from the follicle.

Oestrogens are transported in the blood bound to sex-hormone-binding globulin (SHBG) and albumin. They act via intracellular receptors in the target cells. Oestrogens act on the anterior pituitary and hypothalamus to provide feedback which regulates the system. This feedback is usually negative, but high concentrations of oestrogens for prolonged periods result in a switch to the positive feedback required to induce the LH surge. The actions of oestrogens are shown in Figure 11.7. The main actions are:

- Development of the reproductive organs and secondary sexual characteristics
- Proliferation of the functional layer of uterus endometrium
- Production of watery cervical mucus to allow sperm penetration
- Production of glycogen by the vaginal epithelium.

Progestogens

Progestogens are secreted in the second half of the menstrual cycle by the corpus luteum. This structure is formed by the transformation of the granulosa and theca interna cells in the follicle after ovulation; LH maintains the secretory activity of these cells. The main progestogen is progesterone, which is synthesized from cholesterol in just two steps. During pregnancy, progesterone production is taken over by the placenta.

Progesterone is transported in the blood bound to corticosteroid-binding globulin (CBG) and albumin. It acts via intracellular receptors in the target cells. Progesterone acts on the anterior pituitary and the hypothalamus to provide negative feedback. The actions of progesterone are shown in Figure 11.7. Its main actions are:

- Maintenance of the uterine endometrium
- Stimulation of uterine secretions
- Production of viscid cervical mucus to form an impenetrable barrier.

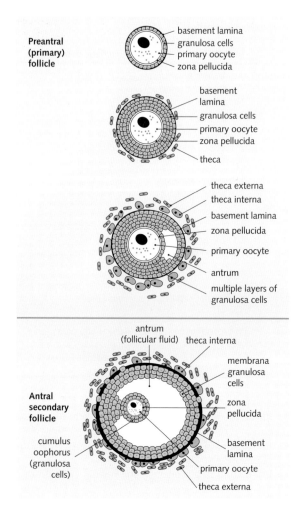

Preantral (primary) follicle
- basement lamina
- granulosa cells
- primary oocyte
- zona pellucida

- basement lamina
- granulosa cells
- primary oocyte
- zona pellucida
- theca

- theca externa
- theca interna
- basement lamina
- zona pellucida
- primary oocyte
- antrum
- multiple layers of granulosa cells

Antral secondary follicle

cumulus oophorus (granulosa cells)

- antrum (follicular fluid)
- theca interna
- membrana granulosa cells
- zona pellucida
- basement lamina
- primary oocyte
- theca externa

Fig. 11.5   Development of an ovarian follicle.

Androgens

The androgens are precursors of oestrogens; however, small quantities are released systemically. They act with adrenal androgen to promote pubic and axillary hair growth during puberty.

Control of ovarian steroid production

Ovarian steroids are regulated in a similar manner to many other major hormones (as shown in Fig. 11.2). Gonadotrophin-releasing factor (GnRH) is synthesized by the hypothalamus and transported to the anterior pituitary gland in the portal veins. Here, it acts on gonadotroph cells to stimulate the release of gonadotrophins (i.e. LH and FSH). This process is described in more detail in Chapter 2.

Gonadotrophins reach the ovaries in the blood and stimulate the release of the ovarian sex steroids. Both LH

and FSH stimulate enzymes involved in oestrogen synthesis. LH also allows the formation and maintenance of the corpus luteum that synthesizes progestogens and oestrogens.

Oestrogens and progestogens feed back to the anterior hypothalamus to regulate their release. This feedback is usually inhibitory and it prevents excess secretion. Before ovulation, the oestrogen feedback becomes positive, triggering the surge in LH release that causes ovulation.

THE MENSTRUAL CYCLE

The menstrual cycle is the process by which the female prepares for possible fertilization of the secondary oocyte. The system is driven by feedback loops between hypothalamic GnRH pulses, pituitary LH and FSH release and ovarian oestrogen, progesterone, inhibin and activin release. Unless interrupted by pregnancy or pathology, these feedback loops generate a cycle that lasts 28–32 days and begins on the first day of menstruation (also called a 'period'). A number of changes occur in the ovaries and endometrium; these are regulated by hormones. The hormonal, ovarian and endometrial changes are shown in Fig. 11.8.

The cycle is divided into two stages, each lasting about 14 days. Between these stages (about the 14th day) ovulation occurs.

Regulation of the cycle by the hypothalamic–pituitary axis

GnRH neurons in the hypothalamus intrinsically generate pulsatile GnRH release. FSH and LH act through endogenous opioids in the hypothalamus to modulate GnRH pulse frequency and amplitude. In turn, the amplitude and frequency of GnRH release dictates the pattern of LH and FSH transcription and release from the pituitary. LH then promotes androstenedione production in the theca cells and FSH stimulates oestrogen production in the granulosa cells and follicular growth.

The first half of the cycle

The first half of the cycle begins on the first day of menstruation and lasts until ovulation. The length of the first half of the cycle is variable; if a woman has a long cycle it is the first stage that is prolonged.

Ovarian changes

This stage of the cycle is called the follicular stage in the ovary.

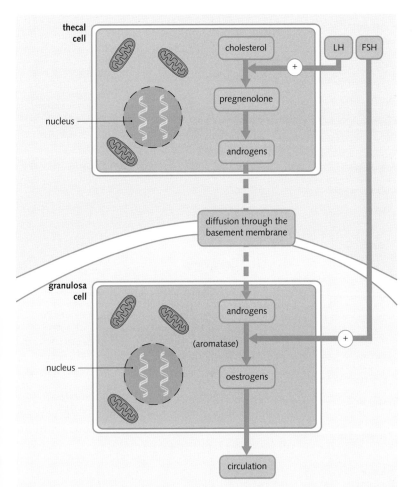

Fig. 11.6 Synthesis of oestrogens by the developing follicle. (FSH, follicle-stimulating hormone; LH, luteinizing hormone.)

During menstruation, LH and FSH levels rise as oestrogen and progesterone production subside. As its name implies, FSH stimulates several antral (secondary) follicles to mature. Cell cooperation between the granulosa cells and the thecal cells allows oestrogen production to begin and for the next 12 days oestrogen levels rise exponentially. Most of the oestrogen output is from the dominant follicle.

The oestrogens stimulate synthesis of LH receptors in the granulosa cells and growth accelerates. With the LH surge, usually only one follicle will be released (the dominant follicle). The other follicles regress (a process called atresia).

Oral contraceptives: administration of synthetic oestrogen and/or progestogen through the first half of the menstrual cycle prevents FSH secretion. This prevents follicular growth so that ovulation cannot occur.

The dominant follicle has a diameter of about 2.5 cm just before ovulation. The development of the follicle is shown in Fig. 11.5. It is composed of seven layers. From the inside out these are as follows:

- Primary oocyte – the female gamete, arrested in first meiotic prophase
- Zona pellucida – a glycoprotein layer that surrounds the oocyte like an egg shell
- Granulosa cells – cuboidal cells surrounding the oocyte; they secrete oestrogens
- Antrum – fluid-filled cavity within the granulosa cells
- Basement membrane/lamina
- Theca interna – a layer of stromal cells that secrete androgens
- Theca externa – a non-secretory stromal cell layer.

Endometrial changes

The first half of the cycle is separated into two phases:

- Menstrual phase
- Proliferative phase.

Fig. 11.7 Actions of oestrogens and progesterone.

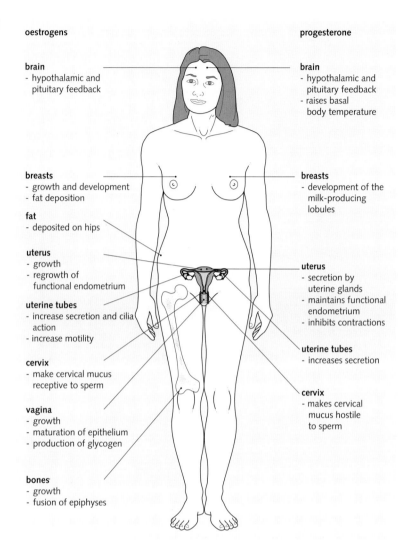

oestrogens

brain
- hypothalamic and pituitary feedback

breasts
- growth and development
- fat deposition

fat
- deposited on hips

uterus
- growth
- regrowth of functional endometrium

uterine tubes
- increase secretion and cilia action
- increase motility

cervix
- make cervical mucus receptive to sperm

vagina
- growth
- maturation of epithelium
- production of glycogen

bones
- growth
- fusion of epiphyses

progesterone

brain
- hypothalamic and pituitary feedback
- raises basal body temperature

breasts
- development of the milk-producing lobules

uterus
- secretion by uterine glands
- maintains functional endometrium
- inhibits contractions

uterine tubes
- increases secretion

cervix
- makes cervical mucus hostile to sperm

During the menstrual phase (days 1–4) the ischaemic and necrotic functional layer of the endometrium is lost. This sloughed tissue passes out of the vagina, along with blood from the degenerating spiral arteries.

The proliferative phase (days 4–13) is caused by the rising oestrogen levels. These stimulate cells in the basal layer of the endometrium to proliferate and form a new functional layer. Glands are formed in this layer but they are not yet active.

The rising oestrogen also stimulates secretion of a watery cervical mucus that facilitates sperm transport across the cervix. At other times, the mucus is scant and thick.

Ovulation

At the end of the follicular stage, the dominant antral follicle secretes such large quantities of oestrogen that the feedback to the pituitary gland changes. The feedback turns from negative to positive and the very high oestrogen levels cause a dramatic surge in the release of LH and, to a lesser extent, FSH. LH causes the follicle to complete the first meiotic division and rupture through the germinal epithelium – a process called ovulation. The secondary oocyte and its first polar body are released into the peritoneal cavity; they are surrounded by the zona pellucida and a few granulosa cells. The released oocyte is swept into the uterine tubes by the wafting action of the cilia of the fimbriae.

The second half of the cycle

The second half of the cycle is the time between ovulation and menstruation; the average length is 14 days and this remains constant despite changes in cycle length. The length is determined by the lifespan of the corpus luteum (about 10 days). This stage of the cycle is called the luteal stage in the ovary.

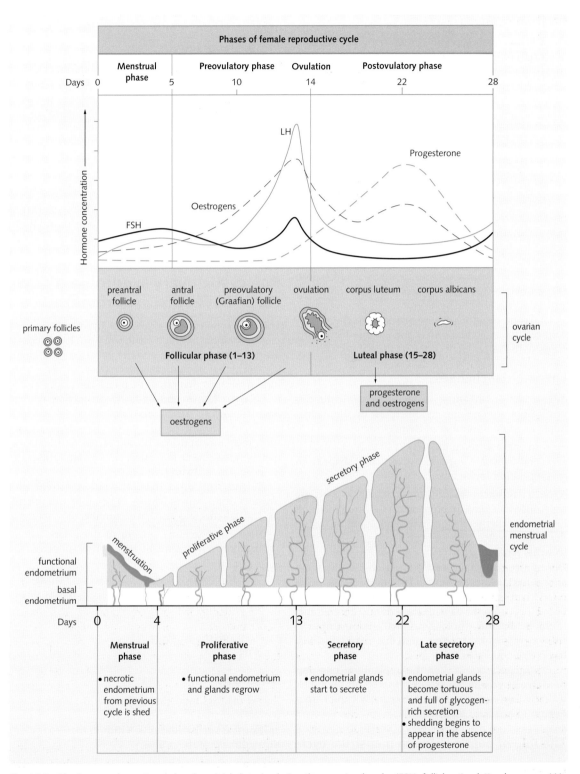

Fig. 11.8 The hormonal, ovarian and endometrial changes during the menstrual cycle. (FSH, follicle-stimulating hormone; LH, luteinizing hormone.)

Ovarian changes

The LH surge continues to act on the granulosa and theca cells in the empty follicle once ovulation has occurred. The cells change and become yellow. They are now called lutein cells (lutein means yellow, hence the name 'luteinizing' hormone) and the rump of the ruptured follicle is called the corpus luteum.

Over the next 10 days, these cells secrete high levels of progesterone and oestrogens, but they then spontaneously involute (shrink) and lose their secretory ability unless they are rescued by the signal of human chorionic gonadotrophin (hCG) produced by the implanting conceptus.

The progesterone and oestrogen secreted by the corpus luteum inhibit LH and FSH release from the pituitary gland. The falling LH levels fail to maintain the corpus luteum, so it undergoes involution. As a result, progesterone and oestrogen levels fall dramatically so their negative feedback to the pituitary gland is lost. FSH and LH secretion rise, causing ovarian follicles to grow, thus starting the next cycle.

Oral contraceptives: the use of oestrogen and/or progestogen in oral contraceptives aims to mimic the early stages of the second half of the menstrual cycle.

Endometrial changes

After ovulation, the progesterone secretion by the corpus luteum activates the endometrium by stimulating differentiation. A number of changes occur:

- Nutrients are stored in the cells
- Glands become tortuous (irregularly shaped) in preparation for secretion.

About 5 days after ovulation, the glands begin to secrete a glycogen-rich 'milk' in preparation for a potential embryo; as a result the changes to the endometrium during the second half of the menstrual cycle are called the secretory phase.

As progesterone and oestrogen levels fall, the spiral arteries supplying the functional endometrium begin to coil and constrict, causing ischaemia and necrosis. Blood leaks from the damaged vessels into the endometrium before the whole functional endometrium is shed. Menstruation occurs, and this marks the first day of the next cycle.

If pregnancy occurs then the implanting conceptus produces hCG, which binds to LH receptors on the luteal cells exerting a luteotrophic signal for the corpus luteum to maintain itself.

The role of peptides in the menstrual cycle

FSH controls the production of inhibin and activin in the granulosa cells. Inhibin A suppresses FSH release during the early follicular phase and inhibin B suppresses FSH during the late phase. Activin facilitates the release of FSH and enhances its actions.

Other ovarian hormones

Inhibin and activin

Inhibin and activin are polypeptide hormones secreted by the granulosa cells of the ovarian follicles. Inhibin inhibits pituitary FSH secretion, while activin stimulates FSH secretion and inhibits androgen production but stimulates conversion to oestrogens. Together, they regulate FSH secretion and local sex steroid levels and the balance between oestrogens and androgens.

Relaxin

This is a polypeptide hormone secreted by the corpus luteum and placenta. It prepares the body for childbirth by causing cervical softening and relaxation of pelvic ligaments.

Polycystic ovary syndrome (PCOS/Stein–Leventhal syndrome)

This is a syndrome composed of hyperandrogenism, oligo-ovulation and polycystic ovaries. The polycystic ovaries must be in the absence of other conditions, e.g. congenital adrenal hyperplasia (late onset) or Cushing's syndrome, that can cause them. The exact cause of PCOS is not known and while it is often familial, there have been no genes yet linked to it.

Patients with this condition often have associated insulin resistance and hyperinsulinaemia, and diabetes/metabolic syndrome may appear as a complication later in those patients who are obese.

Patients with this condition typically present with irregular or infrequent periods or possibly with infertility. The patients may also have a number of other signs:

- Hirsutism (excessive growth of thick dark hair in an androgen-dependent pattern) usually over the upper lip
- Male-pattern baldness
- Acanthosis nigricans (darkened, thick velvety skin in the body folds, usually the neck)
- Obesity
- Deep voice
- Acne.

Diagnosis

Raised LH:FSH ratio (approximately 3:1) with raised testosterone and prolactin. Ultrasound scan will show at least five small follicles, < 5 mm in diameter, along the periphery of the ovaries.

Management

It is necessary to exclude other conditions first. Advice on weight loss and exercise to improve periods and insulin resistance must be given once diagnosis is confirmed. Pharmacologically, metformin is recommended in women of BMI > 25 trying to conceive because of the improvement in insulin sensitivity, ovulatory function and menstrual disturbance. Also available is clomifene, which can stimulate ovulation but increases risks of ovarian cancer. Additionally, the use of ovarian drilling (diathermy creates holes in the ovaries to reduce steroid production) is useful both as a primary treatment of infertility or when clomifene does not work. The combined oral contraceptive pill is found to provide relief of irregular bleeding and can help to reverse the increase in risk of endometrial cancer.

Complications

Patients with PCOS are seen to have increased risk of both endometrial and ovarian cancer. Infertility and hypertension are also known associated problems.

THE MALE REPRODUCTIVE SYSTEM

The male reproductive system consists of five main components (Fig. 11.9):

- Testes – produce the sperm
- Epididymis – stores and matures the sperm
- Vas (ductus) deferens – transports sperm from the epididymis to the penis

- Prostate and seminal vesicles – secrete seminal fluid to support ejaculated sperm
- Penis – deposits sperm in the vagina.

The blood supply, lymphatics and innervation of the male reproductive organs are shown in Fig. 11.10.

Hormones

Testicular sex steroids

The testes secrete 95% of the male sex steroids called androgens; the adrenal cortex is responsible for the remaining 5%. The main androgen is testosterone.

Testicular androgens are secreted by the interstitial Leydig cells found between the seminiferous tubules. They convert cholesterol into the steroid testosterone by a series of reactions. The Leydig cells also secrete small quantities of oestrogens and progestogens as by-products of testosterone synthesis.

Testosterone is a strong androgen. However, some target tissues can convert it to the more potent form called dihydrotestosterone (DHT). The conversion requires the 5-alpha reductase enzyme and occurs in the:

- Sertoli cells
- Prostate gland
- Skin.

Testosterone is transported in the plasma by sex-hormone-binding globulin (SHBG) or albumin. It acts

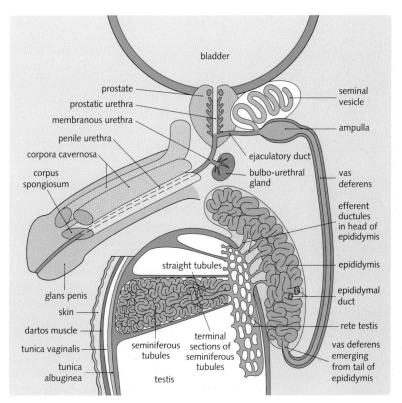

Fig. 11.9 Arrangement of the male reproductive system. This diagram is not to scale.

Fig. 11.10 Blood supply, lymphatics and innervation of the male reproductive organs

Organ	Arterial supply	Venous drainage	Innervation	Lymphatic drainage
Testis	Testicular arteries from the aorta via the spermatic cord	Pampiniform plexus, which forms the testicular veins. Left drains into the left renal vein, right into the inferior vena cava	Sympathetic innervation via the splanchnic nerves	Para-aortic lymph nodes
Scrotum	Pudendal arteries	Scrotal veins	Branches of the genitofemoral, ilioinguinal and pudendal nerves	Superficial inguinal lymph nodes
Prostate	Vesicular and rectal branches of the internal iliac artery	Prostatic venous plexus drains into the internal iliac veins	Parasympathetic via splanchnic nerves; sympathetic from inferior hypogastric plexus	Internal iliac and sacral lymph nodes
Penis	Internal pudendal arteries	Venous plexus, which joins the prostatic venous plexus	Branches of the pudendal nerve	Superficial inguinal lymph nodes

via intracellular receptors to regulate protein synthesis, producing the actions shown in Fig. 11.11. The main actions are:

- Growth and development of the male reproductive tract
- Development of male secondary sexual characteristics (e.g. male hair pattern, muscle growth)
- Stimulation of spermatogenesis
- Stimulation of growth and the fusion of the growth plates of the long bones.

Fig. 11.11 Actions of testosterone

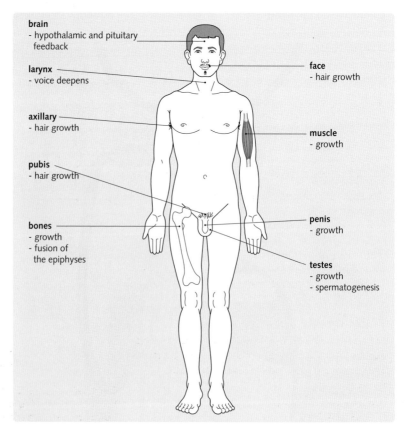

brain
- hypothalamic and pituitary feedback

larynx
- voice deepens

axillary
- hair growth

pubis
- hair growth

bones
- growth
- fusion of the epiphyses

face
- hair growth

muscle
- growth

penis
- growth

testes
- growth
- spermatogenesis

Control of testicular steroid production

Testosterone synthesis and release is controlled by the same hormones in the male as oestrogen synthesis in the female. Gonadotrophin-releasing hormone (GnRH) from the hypothalamus is transported to the anterior pituitary gland by the portal veins. It stimulates the gonadotroph cells to secrete gonadotrophins (LH and FSH). This process is described in more detail in Chapter 2.

LH acts on the Leydig cells to stimulate the first step in testosterone production. Testosterone feeds back to the hypothalamus and pituitary gland to inhibit LH release, but it has little effect on FSH.

FSH acts on the Sertoli cells; it increases the number of testosterone receptors to stimulate spermatogenesis. It also causes inhibin B release from the Sertoli cells, which feeds back to the hypothalamus and pituitary gland to inhibit further FSH release. Inhibin has little effect on LH and therefore regulates sperm production without inhibiting testosterone levels.

Other testicular hormones

The fetal Sertoli cells produce the Müllerian inhibiting substance. This hormone prevents development of the female internal genitalia by causing the Müllerian ducts to regress.

Gynaecomastia

The male breast contains the same tissue components as the female breast in the undeveloped, prepubescent state. If the male breast enlarges, the condition is known as gynaecomastia. It can be defined as the presence of >2 cm of palpable, firm, subareolar gland and ductal breast tissue.

It is caused by any condition or process that raises oestrogen or lowers testosterone levels. It can often occur in puberty, but will usually resolve with time. The underlying cause should be treated if it fails to resolve. Common causes include:

- Oestrogen-containing products or oestrogen-like compounds, e.g. opiates or anabolic steroids
- Hypogonadism or complete gonadal failure; this results in an increase in the oestrogen:testosterone ratio
- Hyperthyroidism and liver cirrhosis can lead to increased synthesis of oestrogens from androstenedione
- Adrenal and testicular tumours.

Investigations

A clear history will help point to the appropriate investigation but in the absence of a clear cause, general investigations can be undertaken. These include:

- FBC/ESR
- U&Es for renal disease
- LFTs to look for liver disease

- TFTs
- CXR, to look for tumours.

The next line of investigation would be to check LH, FSH, oestrogen and testosterone levels. If these tests indicate any abnormalities, further investigations are required. Some specific investigations include:

- Mammography
- Chromosome analysis – Klinefelter's syndrome
- β human chorionic gonadotrophin (hCG), alpha-fetoprotein (AFP) – testicular tumour
- Basal serum prolactin – prolactinoma
- CT head – pituitary tumour.

SOURCES OF REPRODUCTIVE HORMONES

Endocrine signals are essential for implantation and the maintenance of pregnancy. As the pregnancy progresses, the hormone levels change, as shown in Fig. 11.12. There are two phases of hormonal secretion during pregnancy:

- Corpus luteum phase – the corpus luteum secretes hormones to maintain the endometrium and the developing placenta
- Placental phase – the placenta takes over hormonal secretion to allow maternal adaptation to pregnancy, birth and lactation.

Corpus luteum phase

In the normal menstrual cycle, the corpus luteum secretes progesterone and oestrogen for about 10 days following ovulation, after which it regresses. The dramatic fall

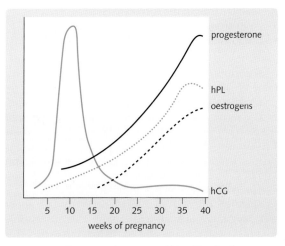

Fig. 11.12 Changes in the maternal blood levels of hormones during pregnancy. (Adapted from D Llewellyn-Jones, 6th edn.)

in progesterone levels causes degeneration and shedding of the endometrium, resulting in menstruation. The blastocyst must prevent the next menstruation by maintaining the corpus luteum and its steroid secretion.

Soon after implantation, around day 6, the syncytiotrophoblast (outer layer of cells) secretes the hormone human chorionic gonadotrophin (hCG). This hormone is equivalent to LH, and it acts on the corpus luteum to prevent regression. Progesterone levels continue to rise and the functional endometrium is maintained. The corpus luteum continues to be the main source of progesterone and oestrogen for the first 6 weeks of development.

Placental phase

The placenta secretes the following hormones:

- hCG
- Progesterone
- Oestrogens
- Human placental lactogen (hPL)
- Relaxin.

Other hormones include placental GnRH, placental CRH, placental TRH, placental ACTH, placental inhibin and placental GH.

By the sixth week the placenta is the main source of progesterone and oestrogens, which help the mother's body adapt to pregnancy. hPL helps regulate nutrient levels and metabolism; it also causes the glandular tissue of the breast to develop. Relaxin is secreted towards the end of pregnancy to prepare the body for birth.

Human chorionic gonadotrophin

hCG is a peptide hormone secreted by the syncytiotrophoblast of the conceptus from implantation. It has a similar structure and actions to LH. These actions include:

- Maintenance of the corpus luteum
- Regulation of placental oestrogen secretion
- Stimulation of testosterone secretion in the male fetus.

The corpus luteum is initially formed and maintained by the ovulatory LH surge and hCG simply replaces the falling levels of LH to prevent regression. hCG is secreted for the first 10 weeks of pregnancy until the placenta is capable of secreting sufficient sex steroids to maintain the pregnancy. After 8 weeks the corpus luteum is no longer needed for hormone production and hCG levels begin to fall.

The β-subunit of hCG can be detected in the urine just before the first day of a missed period, usually about 6–8 days after potential fertilization. This allows time for the blastocyst to implant and hCG levels to rise. This principle is used for the urine pregnancy testing available in hospitals and over the counter in pharmacies. Since hCG levels fall after the corpus luteal phase these tests no longer work after 20 weeks. False positives may rarely indicate underlying disease (see the section on placental disorders).

Progesterone

Plasma levels of progesterone rise throughout pregnancy, secreted initially by the corpus luteum and then by the placenta. It is the single most important hormone in the maintenance of pregnancy. Actions include:

- Maintenance and development of the functional endometrium
- Inhibition of smooth muscle in the uterus to prevent premature expulsion
- Metabolic changes, including fat storage
- Physiological adaptation to pregnancy
- Relaxation of smooth muscle throughout the body, which may cause some side effects (e.g. constipation and oesophageal reflux).

Oestrogens

Plasma levels of oestrogens (especially oestriol) rise throughout pregnancy, secreted initially by the corpus luteum and then by the placenta. Like the granulosa cells, the placenta lacks several key enzymes for the synthesis of oestrogen from cholesterol. These steps must be performed by the fetal adrenal gland, allowing the fetus to regulate placental oestrogen secretion. This does not affect progesterone secretion, which is formed from cholesterol in just two steps.

The actions of oestrogen prepare the body for birth and lactation. They include:

- Growth of the smooth muscle of the uterus (myometrium)
- Increased blood flow to the uterus
- Softening of the cervix and pelvic ligaments
- Stimulation of breast growth and development directly
- Stimulation of pituitary prolactin secretion
- Inhibition of pituitary LH and FSH secretion
- Stimulation of synthesis of oxytocin receptors in the myometrium in late pregnancy
- Water retention.

Human placental lactogen

hPL is a peptide hormone secreted by the syncytiotrophoblast; levels rise throughout pregnancy. It is sometimes called human chorionic somatomammotropin because its actions are similar to growth hormone and prolactin. These actions include:

- Maternal lipolysis (fat breakdown) and fatty acid metabolism sparing glucose
- Maternal insulin resistance sparing glucose for the fetus

- Enhancing active amino acid transfer across the placenta
- Stimulating the growth and development of the breasts
- Increasing cell growth and protein synthesis.

Relaxin

Relaxin is a peptide hormone secreted by the placenta late in pregnancy. It relaxes the myometrium, cervix and the pelvic ligaments, allowing the uterus to enlarge and the pelvis to stretch during birth. It acts by stimulating collagenase enzymes, which break down collagen in these tissues.

REPRODUCTIVE HORMONES FROM OTHER SOURCES

Inhibin

Inhibin is a peptide hormone secreted by the ovary in the pregnant and non-pregnant state. It may suppress pituitary FSH secretion and stimulate progesterone production during pregnancy.

Prolactin

The structure, synthesis and control of prolactin is described in Chapter 2. Prolactin secretion from the pituitary gland rises throughout pregnancy due to stimulation by oestrogens. It has a similar action to hPL in that it stimulates the growth and development of the breasts and regulates fat metabolism.

During pregnancy the high levels of placental oestrogens prevent the secretion of milk. After birth the fall in oestrogen levels allows prolactin to act on the breast. If the mother breastfeeds the baby, sensory signals from the nipple cause further prolactin secretion after pregnancy. The high prolactin levels have two effects:

- Secretion of milk, though it is oxytocin that causes the milk to be ejected
- Inhibition of pituitary FSH and LH, which has a contraceptive effect.

OTHER HORMONAL CHANGES IN PREGNANCY

The secretion of the anterior pituitary hormones is altered during pregnancy (Fig. 11.13):

- FSH and LH secretion is almost completely stopped
- Prolactin secretion rises throughout pregnancy
- Thyroid-stimulating hormone (TSH) secretion initially falls then increases

- Adrenocorticotrophic hormone (ACTH) secretion increases
- Melanocyte-stimulating hormone (MSH) secretion increases.

The anterior pituitary gland enlarges as a result of these changes.

The rise in secretion of most hormones is caused by direct actions of placental hormones and an increase in plasma binding proteins (caused by the action of oestrogens on the liver) that reduces negative feedback.

Thyroid glands

hCG is structurally similar to TSH and inhibits TSH secretion in the first trimester but, as the hCG levels fall in the second and third trimesters, TSH then rises above normal. The increase in TSH, together with a reduction in iodine from the overactive kidneys, causes the thyroid gland to enlarge to trap sufficient iodine. Pregnancy is a state of relative maternal iodine deficiency. Thyroid hormone synthesis also increases but so does the synthesis of thyroid-hormone-binding proteins stimulated by oestrogen. Overall, maternal active/free thyroid hormone levels remain normal. The fetal thyroid secretes thyroxine from 12 weeks; this is independent of maternal control as TSH does not cross the placenta.

Adrenal glands

In contrast, free cortisol levels do rise, despite the increase in plasma-binding proteins. This raises amino acid and glucose levels in the blood to improve fetal growth.

Aldosterone secretion from the adrenal cortex also rises slowly in response to the rising ACTH levels. It helps prevent the sodium loss caused by the raised GFR in the kidney.

Changes in metabolism

The mother usually gains 9–15 kg during pregnancy, though the majority of this is caused by the fetus, placenta and fluid retention. Six months after birth, maternal weight is usually just 1 kg higher than before the pregnancy. Women have a larger appetite during pregnancy to supply the developing fetus, placenta and breasts. The excess of nutrients is regulated by changes in metabolism.

Carbohydrates

The hormone hPL causes insulin resistance to develop by stimulating insulin-like growth factor and this effect is enhanced by the raised cortisol. Insulin production is nearly doubled. The renal threshold for glucose falls and most pregnant women will lose glucose in the urine (glycosuria). As a result, the maternal metabolism uses a higher proportion of fatty acids and glucose use decreases. Pregnancy is a state of progressive insulin resistance due to hPL. This glucose is spared for the growing fetus.

If the mother already has a degree of impaired glucose tolerance (e.g. obesity), then diabetes mellitus can result. The glucose levels should be strictly controlled because hyperglycaemia predisposes to large babies, difficult births and other paediatric complications. After birth, this gestational diabetes mellitus usually resolves.

Amino acids

Progesterone inhibits the breakdown of amino acids in the liver to increase their availability for the fetus. The raised cortisol also increases the blood levels while hPL aids transport across the placenta.

Fat

Fat stores are initially broken down through the action of hPL to drive maternal metabolism. Towards the end of pregnancy, fat is stored in the breasts and subcutaneous tissues. Fat only accounts for a fraction of weight gain through pregnancy.

HORMONAL CONTROL OF PARTURITION

Oxytocin

Oxytocin is a peptide hormone synthesized in the hypothalamus and secreted by the posterior pituitary gland (it is described in Chapter 2).

During labour, oxytocin levels rise due to cervical stimulation by the head. It stimulates uterine contractions that push the fetus against the cervix, stimulating further oxytocin release. A positive feedback mechanism develops called the Ferguson reflex.

Oxytocin receptors in the uterine muscle are increased during late pregnancy by the action of oestrogen. Oxytocin binding stimulates prostaglandin production, which causes the increased contractility (especially PGE_2) and potentiates ion channels, which allow the reflux of Ca^{2+} and Na^+. Stimulation of receptors by oxytocin may also lead to an increase in intracellular Ca^{2+} from sarcoplasmic reticulum.

Prostaglandins

Prostaglandins are locally acting eicosanoids that regulate many processes throughout the body (see Chapter 1). During labour, the prostaglandin PGE_2 is

Fig. 11.13 Changes that occur in pituitary hormone secretion during pregnancy and the effects caused by these changes

Secretion of anterior pituitary hormone	Hormone secretion in pregnancy (compared with non-pregnancy)	Effect of altered plasma hormone level in pregnancy
Prolactin ↑↑↑	Enhanced by placental oestrogens	Promotes growth and development of the breasts and regulates fat metabolism
FSH ↓ and LH ↓	FSH secretion is suppressed by inhibin and placental oestrogens LH secretion is suppressed by the combined effect of progesterone and oestrogen	Prevents further follicular development and ovulation during pregnancy
GH ↓	Suppressed by hPL	Unknown (hPL has similar effect to GH)
ACTH ↑	Rise	Stimulates increased cortisol secretion from the adrenal cortex
TSH	Falls in first trimester but then rises in second and third	Changes in thyroid hormone secretion are counteracted by changes in plasma protein synthesis

ACTH, adrenocorticotrophic hormone; FSH, follicle-stimulating hormone; GH, growth hormone; hPL, human placental lactogen; LH, luteinizing hormone; TSH, thyroid-stimulating hormone.

synthesized in the uterine muscle cells in response to oxytocin. It increases gap junctions and stimulates the release of calcium ions, which cause muscle contractions in a similar fashion to oxytocin.

PGE$_2$ is also synthesized in the cervix, where it stimulates cervical softening and dilatation, known as ripening.

Relaxin

Relaxin promotes the relaxation of the pelvic ligaments and softens the cervix prior to parturition. This allows both structures to stretch so the fetus can pass through the pelvis.

HORMONES AND LACTATION

Lactation is caused by the effects of two hormones:
- Prolactin – causes milk secretion
- Oxytocin – causes milk ejection.

Both hormones are secreted by the pituitary gland in response to nipple stimulation. Prolactin is secreted by the anterior pituitary gland, with production increased by frequent suckling, and oxytocin is secreted by the hypothalamus and released from the posterior pituitary. The synthesis and secretion of these hormones are described in Chapter 2.

Prolactin

Prolactin secretion increases throughout pregnancy, causing the acinar cells of the breast to develop. During pregnancy, milk production is inhibited by high oestrogen levels. After childbirth, oestrogen levels fall dramatically and prolactin stimulates the secretion of milk.

During breastfeeding, stimulation of the nipple causes prolactin secretion, resulting in milk secretion and maintenance of the breast. The milk accumulates within the breast, causing swelling unless oxytocin triggers the milk to be ejected. This neuroendocrine reflex is shown in Fig. 11.14. Once breastfeeding is stopped, nipple stimulation diminishes so prolactin secretion and milk production cease.

The high levels of prolactin during lactation inhibit LH and FSH secretion, giving breastfeeding a contraceptive effect. This is only effective while the baby is suckling regularly. Once lactation ceases, the normal ovarian cycle and fertility return within 4–5 weeks.

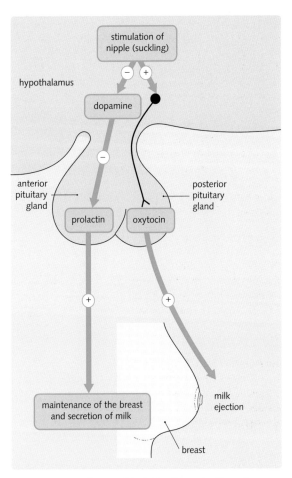

Fig. 11.14   Regulation of lactation by prolactin and oxytocin.

Oxytocin

Milk is ejected from the breast by the action of hormonal, rather than neural, signals on the smooth muscle in the breast. Oxytocin induces the smooth muscle cells surrounding the acini to contract so milk is squeezed out of the nipple. Suckling stimulates this oxytocin release, causing milk ejection within about 30 seconds. The reflex is shown in Fig. 11.14. Even the sound of the baby crying can stimulate the release of oxytocin and the ejection of milk. On the other hand, emotional stress can inhibit this reflex and this can be a particular problem if the woman is worried about her ability to breastfeed.

Self assessment questions

Chapter 2

1. A 51-year-old man presents to A&E with nausea and vomiting. His wife who attends with him remarks that earlier in the day he had a terrible headache, which felt as if he had 'been hit on the head with a baseball bat'. She told him to get some rest and on his way to the door he walked into a coffee table. He has a medical history of hypertension. His current blood pressure is 82/46 mmHg. On inspection the patient appears confused, weak and sweaty. On examination he has a third-nerve palsy and bitemporal hemianopia. What is the most likely diagnosis?
   A. Sheehan's syndrome
   B. Ruptured craniopharyngioma
   C. Pituitary macroadenoma
   D. Pituitary microadenoma
   E. Pituitary apoplexy

2. The patient's blood tests show hypoglycaemia, hypocortisolaemia and low ACTH. What is the most appropriate action?
   A. IV glucose
   B. Transsphenoidal surgery
   C. IV hydrocortisone
   D. Oral prednisolone
   E. IV dexamethasone

3. Which hormone is responsible for the sequelae of Cushing's disease?

   A. ACTH
   B. LH
   C. CRH
   D. Prolactin
   E. Aldosterone

Thyroid Chapter 3

1. A 47-year-old woman presents to her GP concerned about weight loss and diarrhoea she has been experiencing for the last 5 weeks which has gradually worsened. She appears restless throughout the consultation. She says her mother took insulin for diabetes but has no other relevant family history. On examination she was found to be tachycardic (110 bpm) and has a fine tremor in her hands. Exophthalmos and pretibial myxoedema are also noted. The GP orders blood tests for thyroid function but suspects Graves' disease.

Which of the results would be seen if Graves' disease is the cause?

	T$_3$	T$_4$	TSH	Thyroglobulin
A.	Raised	Raised	Raised	Raised
B.	Raised	Raised	Low	Raised
C.	Low	Low	Normal	Normal
D.	Raised	Raised	Low	Low
E.	Raised	Low	Raised	Normal

The presence of thyroid receptor stimulating hormone antibodies (TRAb) is seen in which one of the following?
A. Hashimoto's thyroiditis
B. De Quervain's thyroiditis
C. Graves' disease
D. Primary atrophic hypothyroidism
E. Thyroid hormone resistance syndrome

2. A 34-year-old man presented to A&E with severe heart palpitations and chest pain. The man's history reveals that he was recently at his GP complaining of some mild palpitations, weight loss and agitation. The GP suspected hyperthyroidism and ordered thyroid function tests but the results were not back yet. His wife says he also had a fever and cough over the last few days. On examination, the patient was found to be sweaty and had a tachycardia (approximately 164 bpm) with an irregular rhythm. The patient's mental state has also been deteriorating since he arrived. The doctor suspects a thyroid storm due to the infection.

What is the most appropriate immediate next step with this patient's management?
A. Treatment with β-blocker and carbimazole
B. Treatment with antibiotics for the precipitating infection
C. A technetium scan to confirm thyroid storm
D. Start radioiodine therapy
E. A partial thyroidectomy

What could be another possible precipitant of a thyroid storm in a patient with hyperthyroidism?
A. Cushing's syndrome
B. Recent thyroid surgery
C. A myocardial infarction (heart attack)
D. Hyperglycaemia
E. Excess β-blocker treatment

Adrenal glands Chapter 4

1. A 35-year-old woman was referred to the hospital by her GP with polyuria, polydipsia and altered sensations in her limbs that has been progressively worsening over the last 3 weeks. The hospital rules out type 2 diabetes

but investigations reveal she is hypertensive (154/80 mmHg) as well as hypokalaemic and alkalotic. The doctor diagnoses Conn's syndrome.

What is the cause of Conn's syndrome?
A. Cortisol and aldosterone deficiency
B. ACTH-secreting tumour
C. Adrenaline-secreting tumour
D. Aldosterone-secreting tumour
E. Chronic excessive cortisol secretion

What is the most common cause of secondary hyperaldosteronism?
A. Excessive diuretic therapy
B. Ectopic ACTH secretion
C. Nephritic syndrome
D. Congenital adrenal hyperplasia
E. Acute adrenal cortical failure

2. A 42-year-old male was admitted to the endocrinology ward with increasing weight, central obesity and depression. He also has been having erectile dysfunction for the last month. Cushing's disease is the suspected cause and an overnight dexamethasone suppression test is ordered to confirm.

What is the underlying cause of Cushing's disease?
A. Adrenal adenoma
B. Pituitary adenoma
C. Iatrogenic, i.e. steroid treatment
D. Ectopic ACTH
E. Primary hyperaldosteronism

What is the most appropriate treatment of this disease?
A. An oral glucocorticoid
B. Intramuscular recombinant human growth hormone
C. Stop all current steroid therapy
D. Surgical resection of an underlying tumour
E. An oral angiotensin II receptor blocker

Chapter 6

1. Which of the following is incorrect
   A. GLP-1 enhances insulin release after eating
   B. GLP-1 is degraded by the enzyme DPP-4
   C. GLP-1 is degraded by insulin
   D. Serum leptin levels are higher in people with a greater amount of visceral fat
   E. Low levels of adiponectin are found in people with metabolic syndrome

2. Select the single best answer from the following questions relating to gastrin
   A. Gastrin is secreted in response to fatty acids in the stomach
   B. Gastrin stimulates the release of histamine, which acts on H_1 receptors in the stomach
   C. Gastrin stimulates growth of stomach mucosa and parietal cell maturation
   D. Gastrin stimulates the release of bile from gallbladder
   E. Gastrin causes the pyloric and ileocecal sphincters to contract

3. A 53-year-old man presents to A&E with worsening shortness of breath, palpitations and chest pain over the past 2 hours. He appears sweaty and cyanosed. On examination he has bilateral basal crepitations, left ventricular heave and a displaced apex beat. The doctor suspects congestive heart failure. What blood tests would be used to confirm and assess the severity of heart failure?

A. Troponin T
B. Creatinine kinase cardiac isoenzyme
C. Full blood count
D. Brain natriuretic peptide and NT-pro-BNP
E. Thyroid function tests

Chapter 7

1. A 25-year-old woman presents to her GP with a 2-month history of polydipsia, polyuria and malaise. On further questioning the patient reveals she has not lost any weight, she goes to the toilet approximately once every half an hour and passes large amounts of dilute urine. She has a past medical history of a brain injury that occurred 1 year ago when she was in a road traffic accident. What is the most likely diagnosis?
   A. Type 1 diabetes
   B. Type 2 diabetes
   C. Nephrogenic diabetes insipidus
   D. Neurogenic diabetes insipidus
   E. Pituitary adenoma

2. A 40-year-old man who has been hospitalized with a subarachnoid haemorrhage becomes progressively more confused and agitated. His urinary output is low. Blood tests show hyponatraemia, low plasma osmolality and high urine osmolality. His blood pressure is 130/86 mmHg and he is euvolaemic. What is the most likely diagnosis?
   A. Undiagnosed diabetes
   B. Undiagnosed hypothyroidism
   C. Syndrome of inappropriate ADH secretion
   D. Addison's disease
   E. Acute renal failure

3. ADH has which of following actions?

   A. Increases fluid excretion by inhibiting reuptake of sodium in the distal convoluted tubule
   B. Decreases fluid excretion by increasing sodium uptake in the ascending limb of the loop of Henle
   C. Raises blood pressure by acting on vascular V_2 receptors
   D. Increases water reabsorption in the kidney by acting on V_2 receptors
   E. Is released from the hypothalamus

Chapter 8

1. A 52-year-old woman presents to her GP with a 4-month history of polyuria, polydipsia, depression and malaise. Over the past 2 weeks she has experienced a

dull ache in her right flank which spreads to her abdomen. She thinks this might have a urinary tract infection. Recently, she has felt like her muscles are weak, to the extent that she now finds it difficult to climb stairs. She is currently on hormone replacement therapy. What is the most likely diagnosis?
A. Urinary tract infection
B. Primary hyperparathyroidism
C. Hypoparathyroidism
D. Secondary hyperparathyroidism
E. Hypothyroidism

2. A 67-year-old woman has a bone mineral density (BMD) of >2.5 standard deviations below the mean BMD. She has been advised to stop smoking and given calcium and vitamin D supplements. She has no independent clinical risk factors for fracture. What is the most appropriate pharmacological intervention?
A. Bisphosphonates
B. Teriparatide
C. Calcitonin
D. Strontium ranelate and raloxifene
E. No pharmacological intervention is required

3. Which of the following is an action of parathyroid hormone?
A. Increased excretion of calcium ions from the distal convoluted tubule
B. Increased phosphate reabsorption from the distal convoluted tubule
C. Release of calcium from bone
D. Lowers blood calcium
E. Makes the intestine impermeable to calcium

Pancreas Chapter 5

1. A 45-year-old man was admitted to the emergency department after he was found confused by his family at home. His notes show he has been complaining of headaches and blurred vision for the last 4 months as well as polyuria. He is overweight and you suspect that he has undiagnosed diabetes mellitus type 2.

What would be the most appropriate test to perform to confirm hyperglycaemia in this patient?
A. 2-hour plasma glucose
B. Fasting glucose
C. Glycosylated haemoglobin (HbA1c)
D. Random blood glucose
E. Urine dipstick for glucose

The man is admitted to the ward after successful treatment for hyperglycaemia. The doctor on the ward begins investigations to determine if the man has undiagnosed type 2 diabetes.

What test is necessary to confirm the diagnosis of diabetes?
A. C-peptide level
B. Insulin level

C. Random blood glucose
D. Fasting glucose
E. Glycosylated haemoglobin (HbA1c)

2. A 38-year-old woman presents to her GP with a 2-month history of worsening polyuria and polydipsia. He refers her for investigation, which reveals that she has type 2 diabetes. The GP decides it is necessary to start her on a medication to help manage her condition.

What would be the most appropriate type of medication to use as first-line management in this patient?
A. A thiazolidinedione
B. Subcutaneous insulin
C. A biguanide
D. An incretin mimetic
E. A glyptin
The doctor prescribes metformin for the patient, alongside lifestyle advice for losing weight.

What effect does this drug have on the body?
A. Stimulates β-cells by inhibiting the membrane-bound K^+ channel causing insulin secretion
B. Increases peripheral glucose uptake and reduces glucose output from the liver
C. Increases incretin (GLP-1 and GIP) levels, inhibits glucagon and increases insulin secretion
D. Inhibits intestinal enzymes, preventing the digestion of starch
E. Promotes insulin secretion, reduces glucagon activity and slows glucose absorption from the gut

Growth Chapter 9

1. A 13-year-old boy is referred to see a paediatrician because his parents think he has not started puberty and have noticed he is quite a bit shorter than his peers. He has no distinct medical complaints but is worried about being too small for his school hurling team. The paediatrician examines the boy and says that clinically he has started puberty and is in Tanner's stage 1.

Using Tanner's staging, the testes must be greater than what volume if puberty is said to have started?
A. 4 mL
B. 6 mL
C. 10 mL
D. 16 mL
E. 18 mL

The boy's parents are quite short themselves and the patient is curious about how tall he might grow to. The doctor decides to work out the mean parental height (MPH).

The MPH for the boy is calculated by averaging the parent's heights, then doing what?
A. Subtract 7 cm
B. Subtract 5 cm
C. Add 5 cm
D. Add 7 cm
E. Add 10 cm

Neoplastic syndromes Chapter 10

1. A 29-year-old man is referred to the endocrinology clinic with a 5-week history of unexplained flushing in his face and upper chest. The man has also been experiencing diarrhoea and vomiting that have worsened over time. The man has no family history of any relevant conditions. The doctor examines the patient and notes several murmurs on auscultation that were not previously noted by the man's GP. The doctor suspects cardiac damage secondary to carcinoid syndrome.

If liver metastases are the source of the hormones, damage to which two valves in the heart is associated with carcinoid syndrome?
A. Pulmonary and aortic
B. Pulmonary and tricuspid
C. Aortic and mitral
D. Tricuspid and mitral
E. Pulmonary and mitral

What substance secreted by a carcinoid tumour/metastasis causes the fibrosis in the heart valves?
A. Serotonin
B. Bradykinin
C. Tachykinin
D. Gastrin
E. ACTH
The diagnosis of carcinoid syndrome is confirmed and now the primary tumour must be located for surgical removal.

Outside of the gastrointestinal tract, where can primary carcinoid tumours occur?
A. The heart
B. The brain
C. The lungs
D. The lymph nodes
E. The kidneys

Reproductive hormones Chapter 11

1. A 19-year-old woman presents to her GP complaining she has been unable to get pregnant despite trying for 2 years. The woman has also been having irregular periods since she started puberty. The woman has hirsutism and poorly controlled acne, and her hair has also been getting progressively thinner during the last few weeks. Her family history reveals that her mother is obese and suffers from type 2 diabetes. The patient is 135 cm tall and weighs 62 kg. The GP suspects polycystic ovary syndrome (PCOS) and refers the girl for tests at the hospital.

Which of these hormones is raised in PCOS?
A. Luteinizing hormone
B. Follicle-stimulating hormone
C. Oestradiol
D. Human chorionic gonadotrophin
E. 17-Hydroxyprogesterone
The girl also mentions that she has been having polyuria and polydipsia, so the doctor investigates for diabetes as well. The results of the investigations indicate an impaired fasting glucose, not diabetes.

In a patient with IFG, what would be the 2-hour result seen after investigation with a 2-hour plasma glucose test?
A. 7.0 mmol/L
B. 7.9 mmol/L
C. 8.5 mmol/L
D. 10.6 mmol/L
E. 11.2 mmol/L

What is the most appropriate pharmacotherapy for this patient?
A. Gliclazide
B. Metformin
C. Insulin
D. GLP-1
E. Sitagliptin

Extended-matching questions (EMQs)

For each scenario described below, choose the *single* most likely diagnosis from the list of options. Each answer may be used once, more than once or not at all.

1. The pancreas and diabetes.

A. Type 2 diabetes

B. Gestational diabetes mellitus

C. Hyperosmotic non-ketotic diabetic coma (HONK)

D. Diabetic ketoacidosis

E. The metabolic syndrome

F. Maturity-onset diabetes of the young (MODY)

G. Hypoglycaemia

Instruction: Match the diagnosis to the following clinical scenarios:

1. A 60-year-old women whose recent-onset diabetes is entirely controlled by diet, metformin and sulphonylureas.
2. A 15-year-girl with diabetes who is known to suffer from a mutation in the glucokinase gene.
3. A 50-year-old man suffering from mild fasting hyperglycaemia, hypertriglyceridaemia and central adiposity who has deranged function tests.
4. A 10-year-old boy who is found in his room drowsy, vomiting, severely dehydrated, suffering from acidotic breathing (Kussmal breathing).
5. A 42-year-old pregnant women with hyperglycaemia who has family history of NIDDM and has previously given birth to a large baby.

2. The hypothalamus and the pituitary gland.

A. Supraoptic nucleus

B. Antidiuretic hormone

C. Sheehan's syndrome

D. The syndrome of inappropriate ADH secretion

E. Oxytocin

F. Gonadotrophs

G. Prolactinoma

H. Pars distalis

I. Lactotrophs

J. Pituicytes

Instruction: Match the appropriate letter to the following numbered statements:

1. The cells which produce prolactin.
2. The hormone which does not function appropriately in diabetes insipidus.
3. A common cause of galactorrhoea.
4. A cause of hyponatraemia in a woman suffering from post-partum haemorrhage.
5. The cells which secrete follicle-stimulating hormone

3. The adrenal glands.

A. Phaeochromocytoma

B. Conn's syndrome

C. Renal artery stenosis

D. Cushing's syndrome

E. Congenital adrenal hyperplasia

F. Addison's disease

G. Bartter's syndrome

Instruction: Match the diagnosis to the following clinical scenarios:

1. A 45-year-old woman with buccal hyperpigmentation, weakness, abdominal pain, hyperkalaemia and hypernatraemia.
2. A 36-year-old man with a hypochloremic metabolic alkalosis, low serum renin and a mass in the adrenal glands on MRI.
3. A 30-year-old female who presents with episodic pallor, chest pain and hypertension. A cause of hyponatraemia in a woman suffering from post-partum hemorrhage.
4. A rheumatology patient on long-term steroids who presents with weight increase, moon face, menstrual irregularity and purple striae.
5. A young girl presenting with virilism and hirsutism.

4. Endocrine disease.

A. Cushing's disease

B. Acromegaly

C. Graves' disease

D. Dwarfism

E. Diabetes mellitus

F. Adipsic diabetes insipidus

Instruction: Decide which endocrine disease may be implicated in each of these scenarios:

127

1. A 55-year-old man who presents with a large jaw and bitemporal hemianopia.
2. A 25-year-old woman who presents with excessive micturition who does not become thirsty on hyperosmolar stress testing.
3. A 50-year-old woman with an irregular pulse (i.e. atrial fibrillation), tremor and exophthalmos.
4. A 76-year-old woman with rheumatoid arthritis who presents with depression and a fractured neck of femur.
5. A 63-year-old patient with renal failure, angina and deteriorating sight.

5. Thyroid disease.

A. Thyrotoxicosis
B. Papillary thyroid cancer
C. Myxoedema
D. Hyperthyroidism
E. Ophthalmoplegia
F. Follicular thyroid cancer
G. Adipsic diabetes insipidus

Instruction: Decide which of A–G best matches each of the statements below:

1. A disease of the thyroid which is often associated with the production of a fusion protein.
2. A sign of Graves' disease.
3. A disease of the thyroid which is often associated with activation of the *RET* proto-oncogene.
4. A symptomatic patient with high serum thyroid hormone which is being produced by a struma ovarii.
5. Puffiness on the anterior surface of the lower leg.

6. Symptoms of pregnancy.

A. Rising oestrogen levels
B. Progesterone-induced smooth muscle relaxation
C. Raised serum TSH
D. Oestrogen-induced ligament softening
E. Raised melanocyte-stimulating hormone level
F. Impaired glucose tolerance due to the actions of cortisol

Instruction: Match each of these conditions with the appropriate physiological change from the list above:

1. Gestational diabetes.
2. Morning sickness.
3. Goitre.
4. Back ache.
5. Constipation.

7. Disorders of pregnancy.

A. Placental abruption
B. Placenta praevia
C. Pre-eclampsia
D. Ectopic pregnancy
E. Hydatidiform mole
F. Sheehan's syndrome

Instruction: Match each of these characteristics with the appropriate condition from the list above:

1. A women in the third trimester of her pregnancy presents with high blood pressure, oedema and proteinuria.
2. A pregnant women with pelvic inflammatory disease presents with severe abdominal pain and sudden collapse.
3. A pregnant women with polyhydramnios presents with vaginal bleeding and abdominal pain. Ultrasound reveals serious intrauterine blood clots.
4. A pregnancy in which the placenta is located over the lower uterine segment.
5. A condition in which chorionic villi form grape-like vesicles.

8. Signs of endocrine disease.

A. Acromegaly
B. Cushing's disease
C. Goitre
D. Pituitary tumour
E. Congenital adrenal hyperplasia
F. Infection with *Candida albicans*
G. Hypopituitarism
H. Rickets

Instruction: Match each of these signs or symptoms with the appropriate endocrine disease:

1. Bilateral decrease in breast size.
2. Clitoromegaly.
3. Thick, white, cottage-cheese-like inflammation of the skin and mucous membranes.
4. 'Pigeon' chest.
5. Papilloedema.

9. Signs of endocrine disease.

A. Blood glucose of 7.3 mmol/L 2 hours after glucose intake
B. No cortisol suppression on high-dose dexamethasone suppression test after a positive low-dose test

C. Thyroid-stimulating antibodies in the blood

D. Slight depression of cortisol on high-dose dexamethasone suppression test after a positive low-dose test

E. Fasting blood glucose of 6.5 mmol/L

F. Anti-thyroid peroxidase and anti-thyroglobulin antibodies

Instruction: Match each of these diseases to the appropriate findings on investigation:

1. Hashimoto's thyroiditis.
2. ACTH-secreting tumour.
3. Normal glucose tolerance.
4. Graves' disease.
5. Impaired glucose tolerance.
6. Ectopic ACTH-secreting tumour or adrenal tumour.

10. Imaging and endocrine disease

A. Osteosclerotic lesions

B. Osteolytic lesions

C. Osteoporosis

D. Osteomalacia

E. Enlarged sella turcica

F. Organ calcification

Instruction: Match each of these pathologies with the appropriate bone conditions suggested by X-ray findings from the list above:

1. Prostate bony metastases.
2. Thyrotoxicosis.
3. Pituitary adenoma.
4. Adrenal disease.
5. Hyperparathyroidism.

SAQ answers

SINGLE BEST ANSWERS

Chapter 2
1. E
2. C
3. A

Chapter 3
1. B, C
2. A, B

Chapter 4
1. D, A
2. B, D

Chapter 5
1. D, D
2. C, B

Chapter 6
1. E
2. D
3. D

Chapter 7
1. D
2. C
3. D

Chapter 8
1. D
2. E
3. C

Chapter 9
1. A, D

Chapter 10
1. B, A, C

Chapter 11
1. A, A, B

EMQ answers

1. The pancreas and diabetes

1. A
2. F
3. E
4. D
5. B

2. The hypothalamus and the pituitary gland

1. I
2. B
3. G
4. C
5. F

3. The adrenal glands

1. F
2. B
3. A
4. D
5. E

4. Endocrine disease

1. B
2. F
3. C
4. A
5. E

5. Thyroid disease

1. F
2. E
3. B
4. A
5. C

6. Symptoms of pregnancy

1. F
2. A
3. C
4. D
5. B

7. Disorders of pregnancy

1. C
2. D
3. A
4. B
5. E

8. Signs of endocrine disease

1. G
2. E
3. F
4. H
5. D

9. Signs of endocrine disease

1. F
2. D
3. A
4. C
5. B

10. Imaging and endocrine disease

1. A
2. C
3. E
4. F
5. D

Note: Page numbers followed by *b* indicate boxes, and *f* indicate figures.